Adalberto Llinás Delgado

Integrated health management

Adalberto Llinás Delgado

Integrated health management

ScienciaScripts

Imprint

Cover image: www.ingimage.com

This book is a translation from the original published under ISBN 978-613-9-18902-1.

Publisher:
Sciencia Scripts
is a trademark of
Dodo Books Indian Ocean Ltd. and OmniScriptum S.R.L publishing group

120 High Road, East Finchley, London, N2 9ED, United Kingdom
Str. Armeneasca 28/1, office 1, Chisinau MD-2012, Republic of Moldova, Europe
Managing Directors: Ieva Konstantinova, Victoria Ursu
info@omniscriptum.com

Printed at: see last page
ISBN: 978-620-8-52086-1

Contents

Foreword 4
Chapter 1 5
Chapter 2 14
Chapter 3 23
Chapter 4 34
Chapter 5 39
Chapter 6 58
Chapter 7 76
Chapter 8 87
Chapter 9 111
Chapter 10..114
Chapter 11..119
Chapter 12..126
Chapter 13..138
Chapter 14..146
Chapter 15..153
BIBLIOGRAPHY...158

Authors:
Aleyda Parra Castillo Sandra Gómez Aguirre Kissy Macías Bolívar Pedro Llinás Burgos Gladys Gaviria García Rusvelt Vargas Moranth Adalberto Llinás Delgado

Collaboration of the Nutrition and Public Health Research Seminar.

Adrián Yaseth Vargas López Alejandra Carolina Fontalvo González Andrea Yulidza Stand Muñoz

Camila Johana Zapata Cervera Greydis De la Hoz Manotas Helda Rosa Rivera Muñoz

Jennifer Carolina Mercado Charris

Keila Margarita Fonseca Pérez Keyla Marcela De León Fontalvo Laura Daniela Albor Jiménez

Leidys Paola Sotomayor Salcedo Liliana Marcela Isaza Polo

Luz Divina Diaz Rivera

Maicol David Butajo Noriega

Maria José Castilla Reyes

Nickol Andrea Rivera García

Olga Sofia Caballero López

Valentina Palacín Martínez

Valentina Del Carmen Vargas Romero

Yurainis Paola Ruiz Alvear

Foreword

The past Covid-19 pandemic has come to mean that we must take a break, it is time to reflect and consider new directions in health. It is time to innovate the old Flexnerian model which, despite all its application and success in different countries of the world, is not the solution to the serious public health problems, as has been demonstrated by the strong economic implications worldwide.

With the arrival of the new millennium, which has brought with it new technologies that can be used in medicine, it is imperative to change the health model in all areas, in the sense of moving from a curative model to a predictive one, for which doctors must acquire new competencies, not only in the field of medicine, but also in the field of administration, This means that doctors must acquire new skills, not only in the field of medicine but also in administration, and thus be able to establish an integrated health management system, optimally managing a country's resources, so as not to have to spend enormous economic resources when serious events occur, as has happened in the past, when governments have had to spend what was not budgeted for.

For this reason, the academic document sets out in the following arguments the why, what, where, how, as well as the tools that can be used in order to move towards the implementation of integrated health management in the country, which is urgently needed to fully benefit from 21st century medicine. The country cannot turn its back on the new technological developments that are revolutionising all the concepts of science, where medicine could not become an island, for this is that a vision of the world is required, where medicine not only fulfils its restorative function but quite the opposite, to be able to anticipate so that it does not happen again like the Covid-19 pandemic where, due to lack of foresight and anticipation, many inhabitants of the world had to leave, leaving us all with a lesson to overcome, such as radically changing the way of approaching the study and medical practice after this devastating pandemic.

Chapter 1

A New Challenge

In the society towards which we are rapidly moving, the key resource is knowledge Peter Drucker.

"Plans are useless, but planning is indispensable." Dwight D. Eisenhower

Nobody was talking about a pandemic until a few years ago, the coronavirus came along, and suddenly it changed our lives and forced us to step out of our comfort zone and do things differently. Life in the COVID-19 era is totally new and unexpected, and perhaps none of us would be in a position to claim to be prepared for this situation. The emergency is over, but the virus is still with us. This new challenge allows us to better address emerging diseases among health determinants and prepares us to implement timely and effective response models for the next epidemiological event.

Therefore, one must be prepared to solve social problems where optimal use of resources, which as always are limited and scarce, is required; to achieve this, strategies, policies and procedures are developed in accordance with evolving management concepts and techniques. In his book How to Avoid the Next Pandemic, the famous philanthropist Bill Gates urges us to be fully prepared "We should not assume that the next pandemic threat will be exactly like Covid-19. It will affect young people. The impact may be greater in older adults, or it can also be spread by adhering to surfaces or through human faeces. It may be more contagious and spread more easily from person to person. Or it could be more deadly. Or, worse, it could be more deadly and contagious.

To meet these challenges, integrated health management based on the development of effective health management models from a collective health identity, in dialogue with basic and clinical biomedical sciences, as well as with social, economic, environmental and scientific sciences, is essential. Politics and demography are the current and future challenges of our society. Therefore, health system management competencies and skills are essential to ensure continued growth and efficiency. A health professional may be highly skilled in his or her field, but at the same time may lack specific management experience and training, or be an expert in this field and not be aware of public health issues. Management cannot be the same for all industries, particularly when it comes to health institutions.

Today, people's demand for medical care is very important. This phenomenon is not new, but over time, the number and complexity become obvious, reflecting a long-term dilemma for health institutions and professionals. Health systems must be designed to meet service needs and the resulting social functions. A health system is a well-connected relationship between resources, finance, organisation and management to provide adequate and timely care to the users of the system. Effective management will be able to achieve the goals set out in the various health programmes and thus respond to the needs of society.

The priority of the health system should be to develop the management capacity of those responsible for it. Therefore, the management of health systems requires a set of knowledge, skills, techniques and competencies that form a harmonious balance that prepares the manager and allows him/her to carry out a series of actions to achieve the goals set in the solution of priority problems. In Health Management, it is necessary to have a broad and comprehensive knowledge of the system; therefore, their work goes beyond the management of clinics, hospitals, medical departments or health centres, and in any of these scenarios they must be able to deal with planning, execution, control, monitoring and feedback (PLECOSER), which requires extensive knowledge in the field of health.

An environment where system leadership positions must be filled by professionals trained to make complex decisions, while at the same time it is very difficult to balance fluctuations in scale to achieve a balance between needs and resources. Managers are sometimes unclear about their job role and expectations; therefore, the central idea is the desire to position themselves in a hierarchy without training, focusing only on image or authority. Professional development is the key to success in healthcare management. Healthcare managers must take steps to assess, develop and hone the personal and professional skills essential to maintain their competence.

Most training programmes focus on traditional clinical practice with an emphasis on major diseases, but institutional leaders will be challenged to change this dynamic.

In the future, healthcare managers will need to adopt an approach that involves patients more in self-care; offering alternatives to current practice. Getting staff to interact with patients without consulting them, thus avoiding congestion and overcrowding by reducing the burden on the point of care.

Some authors have questioned who should manage health services. Paradoxically, it is persuasive to say that a health professional is not qualified to lead, although he or she is likely to have the trust and cooperation of all staff and therefore be in a better position to make decisions.

On the other hand, it is mentioned that professionals with specific training in administration who are not linked to the health area have outstanding management skills when holding a managerial position in health care institutions. Without delimiting this controversy, it is clearly necessary to train workers in the sector in administrative competencies with validated models for intervention in the health area so that they can actively participate in decision-making.

We must understand that good administration in the health area is not a panacea that by itself will solve all the problems, but it will allow us to form an organisation with efficient processes, establishing an analytical structure of marked usefulness in the practice of health care in the communities, centred on the quality and humanisation of the services provided.

The implementation of the preventive model is a major challenge that must be faced. In 2010, Dr. Adalberto Llinás, in an article entitled "Evaluation of the quality of health care, a first step for the reform of the system", framed in the immanent need for the right to health as a fundamental principle, suggested "the need to generate models of quality of care centred on the human being, prioritising health without neglecting coverage" ... This reflection suggests "the need to generate models of quality of care centred on the human being, prioritising health without neglecting coverage". This reflection suggests "the need to generate models of quality care centred on the human being, prioritising health without neglecting coverage" ... the creation of "a health model centred on quality is an ethical imperative, which must start from academia, with broad citizen participation". Everything indicates that this reflection could become a reality in Colombia and will undoubtedly be a topic worthy of being explored by the academy.

In this document, the group of researchers from the Faculty of Nutrition and Dietetics of the Universidad del Atlántico propose some lines and concepts to implement a management model that, without seeking to be exclusive or exhaustive, establishes a solid foundation to achieve the implementation of patient-centred health systems, providing timely and efficient care with protocols based on current scientific evidence and with cost-effective investments in individual and collective health, prioritising prevention, primary care and preparation to address current problems effectively and that at the same time can leave us prepared for the future. The model leads to investments that include strengthening primary care centres, investment in laboratories, research, protection of human talent and epidemiological surveillance.

The health reform presented on 13 February 2023 by the national government, in its Article 68, establishes the need for refresher courses in hospital administration every two years for directors of state health institutions. Colombia has a population of around 48.3 million inhabitants according to the

2018 Census, 97% of whom are covered by one of the two mandatory health plans. The subsidised scheme has a membership of more than 23 million people; the contributory scheme has 21 million members and there are an estimated 2.4 million people in the exempted schemes (DANE).
It is necessary to underline that the Colombian population is ageing rapidly and supports a system similar to that of the OECD member countries. The adult population makes up the majority of the population and has a high risk of contracting non-communicable diseases, which is demonstrated by the high number of consultations per person per year. This adult population suffers from many pathologies, which in most cases can be prevented, this is manifested as a minimum percentage, 10% of the population consumes 80% of the health resources.
In terms of distribution, the growth of the population residing in large cities is accelerating. Between 1985 and 2014 it grew by 13%, reaching 76.3% of the Colombian population. It is estimated that by 2050, 85% of the population will reside in Colombia's largest cities.
The Colombian epidemiological profile shows that the leading cause of death in the adult population continues to be ischaemic heart disease, which accounts for 48.16% of deaths, cardiovascular diseases, with 29.69%, are responsible for deaths in adults; Cerebrovascular diseases with 24.07% and complications related to arterial hypertension and similar disorders with 9.97%; neoplasms and external causes were placed as the second and third cause of death in the general population with 17.42% and 17.33% of total mortality respectively.
In men, stomach cancer is the leading cause of death from neoplasms, malignant tumours of the digestive organs and peritoneum, except stomach and colon are the second cause, and the third cause of death is attributed to prostate cancer.
In women, the main cause of death from neoplasms is cancer of the digestive organs and peritoneum, with the exception of the stomach and colon. In second place are malignant tumours of other and undetermined locations, and in third place is breast cancer, with prognoses of constant increase over time.
The study of external causes shows that violent deaths are the leading cause of mortality among men, with the following distribution: homicides account for 53.43% of deaths, road traffic accidents 18.59%, and in third place are suicides.
Mortality due to communicable diseases has been on a downward trend over time, while acute respiratory diseases account for 48.21% of mortality, and deaths due to HIV/AIDS have reached 17.79%.
In turn, high-cost diseases as events of major public health importance directly related to high economic factors, such as end-stage chronic kidney disease,

requiring renal replacement therapy or transplantation, associated with arterial hypertension, diabetes mellitus or both, and whose occurrence has been increasing in the last 5 years.

In addition, obesity in people aged between 18 and 64 years has been rising; its percentage in 2015 was 20% higher than in 2010, changing from 13.70 cases to 16.50 per 100 people. For this population obesity is found in 75% more females than males, with an absolute difference of 8.6 women with greater obesity per 100; being 19% higher in the city than in the countryside, finally, it can occur in 26% more in people without any education, in relation to those with higher education.

On the other hand, about 82% of deaths occurring in children under five years of age are observed before the first year of life and are usually attributed to congenital disorders, respiratory disorders and other pathologies occurring in the perinatal stage, acute respiratory infections and bacterial sepsis. For children between one and four years of age, the high mortality rates are due to external factors whose incidence has been declining from 19.01 in 2005 to 12.86 deaths per 100,000 in 2015.

In the population of children under five years of age, mortality continues, but on the rise, due to diseases such as acute diarrhoea and respiratory diseases. Mortality due to malnutrition continues, with 80% of this prevalence among the 50% of the population with the highest percentage of people with unsatisfied basic needs. There are strong and undesirable differences between the different regions, departments and municipalities , demonstrating difficulties of inequity in health.

In addition to the above, in terms of changes in the epidemiological tables, changes in the socio-cultural environment in Colombia are developing within society, i.e. within the family, variations and difficulties, as well as new family structures or types. In the second half of the 20th century, there was a characteristic increase in the number of de facto marital unions among couples, where family separations have multiplied exponentially in the last 30 years. In this same condition, Colombia has the first place among the countries in the world where children are procreated by couples without formal marital unions; and 50% of the separations of unions involve at least two previous unions. The prevalence of these actions is balanced by the social character of the households and therefore the types of families that are currently being erected in Colombian society.

Likewise, a situation in Colombian households that has been occurring for some decades is the change in the head of household from male to female. In 2000, 25% of heads of household were women, by 2005 this had risen to 28%, and by 2010 it had risen to 30%. By 2015, it had risen to 34%. This demonstrates the increasing trend of the transfer of headship in Colombian households, in which it is women who are in charge. This increase is observed in both large cities and rural areas.

Another issue of great importance for countries is that of mental health. In this regard, at least 40.1% of Colombians have suffered at some time from a mental disorder, primarily anxiety, as a result of a lack of emotional support and the use of psychotropic substances. As a result of the conflict, 20% of the population suffer from some degree of depression, 91% suffer from anxiety and 14% have psychosis; without ignoring the fact that over the last 14 years, a figure of 3,700,381 people and 846,386,381 people have suffered from psychosis.700,381 people and 846,655 families have been displaced; as a product of violence, it has become a public health problem, demonstrating the urgent need to strengthen mental health prevention programmes and therefore integral management programmes within the family.

Another element of great importance for Colombian society according to the report published by the Colombian Association for the Protection of Abused Minors is the increase in social violence, where domestic violence tends to be the most represented. Within this intra-family violence it is possible to establish violence between partners, where the female gender is the main victim, followed by child violence, which is a negative factor for the normal development of the family.

In short, Colombia is lagging behind in defining primary health care guidelines, which could become a cornerstone for the advancement of new training approaches that take into consideration the new information and communication technologies that contribute to promote a holistic approach to health, integrating the biological, environmental and social branches in which life develops, and be able to strengthen the power of resolution at the first levels of care, as well as the continuity and comprehensiveness of the care process. Therefore, the strengthening of family and community medicine programmes, with a focus on primary health care and family health, is currently a real necessity.

It is also worth noting that in order to achieve an efficient health system, the training of human talent must not be ignored. The need for distance education, which became widespread after the pandemic, takes us back to a *Dèjá vu* in the days when teaching was done via national radio, but it is clear that the future of health education with an exclusive face-to-face system has its days numbered. We now know that classrooms that encourage discussion and dialogue among students, as well as collaboration, better activate neuroplasticity and lead to better learning outcomes, so the use of virtuality can lead to greater teacher-student engagement. A pairing for optimal interaction in knowledge sharing.

We hope that this book will contribute to a holistic view of the academic training process, understanding that training produces knowledge, but it must also contribute to the formation of better people.

General Health Administration Students' Contribution to this Chapter

"A New Challenge" is a critical analysis and commentary on the challenges in the health system in Colombia and how to address them in the future. The text covers a wide range of topics related to health management and offers a comprehensive view of the problems and opportunities in this field. Some key points are presented below:

- The pandemic as a turning point: The text begins by highlighting how the COVID-19 pandemic radically changed people's lives and highlights the need to prepare for future epidemiological events. This focus on health crisis preparedness is fundamental and shows an awareness of the importance of health planning and management.
- Integrated health management: Emphasis is placed on the importance of effective, multidisciplinary health system management, encompassing not only medical but also social, economic and environmental aspects. This reflects a deep understanding of the complexity of the health system and the need to address problems from multiple perspectives.
- Training of health professionals: The need to train health professionals in management skills is mentioned, which is essential to ensure an efficient health system. Training should not only be limited to clinical practice, but should also include aspects of administration and management.
- Importance of good governance in health: It is stressed that effective governance will not solve all health problems, but can contribute to efficient processes and quality patient-centred care.
- Specific health problems in Colombia: The text presents relevant data on the health situation in Colombia, including the ageing population, chronic diseases, high mortality rates from cardiovascular diseases and regional disparities in health care. These issues are fundamental to understanding the challenges facing the Colombian health system.
- Preventive model and patient-centred care: The need to adopt a more preventive approach to health care and to involve patients in self-care is mentioned. The aim is to reduce congestion in care facilities.
- Mental health and violence: The importance of addressing mental health problems and violence, which are significant concerns in Colombia, is

highlighted. This reflects an understanding that health is not only limited to physical aspects, but also includes mental and social aspects.

• Health education: The text discusses the need to adapt health education to technological changes and the importance of distance learning. It also emphasises the importance of encouraging discussion and collaboration among students for effective learning.

Overall, "A New Challenge" provides a comprehensive analysis of the health situation in Colombia and outlines key solutions and approaches to address future challenges. It highlights the importance of effective management, training of health professionals in management skills and attention to specific health problems in Colombian society. It also recognises the need to adapt to technological changes in health education to produce more competent and well-rounded professionals.

Questionnaire

d. What is one of the main health challenges in Colombia mentioned in the document?

a) Lack of access to health care
b) Increase in obesity
c) Shortage of health professionals
d) Low quality of health services

Answer: b) Increased obesity

2. What is mentioned as a need in academic training in the health field?

a) Strengthening mental health programmes
b) Improving primary health care
c) Training management professionals
d) Implementing a patient-centred model of care

Answer: c) To train management professionals.

3. What is one of the shortcomings of the document mentioned in the critique?

a) Lack of updated data
b) Absence of specific recommendations
c) Little deepening of distance education
d) Lack of discussion on equity in health care

Response: b) No specific recommendations

4. What is one of the impacts of the pandemic mentioned in the document?

a) Increase in domestic violence
b) Shortage of resources in the health system
c) Increased demand for medical care
d) Decreasing obesity in the population

Answer: c) Increased demand for medical care

5. What is one of the health system management competencies and skills mentioned in the document?

a) Knowledge of basic and clinical biomedical sciences

b) Experience in administration of health institutions

c) Social problem-solving skills

d) Understanding demographic and political challenges

Answer: d) Understanding the demographic and political challenges

Open Questions

1. What specific challenges does health systems management face as expressed in the text?
2. How is it mentioned that domestic violence and mental health are related?
3. Do you think our current health system is prepared for a pandemic or epidemiological crisis?
4. What is the main idea that stands out about the COVID-19 pandemic and its impact on health management?
5. What is the final message of the text in relation to academic health education?

Chapter 2

Formative Model of Knowledge Sharing: Building the Context of a New Post-Pandemic Scenario

Context of a New Post-Pandemic Scenario

Nature has given us the seeds of knowledge, not knowledge itself.

Seneca

The educational process is part of our world. People decide to integrate and change them when they feel frustrated. The philosophy of education provides the theoretical orientation necessary to not get lost in the learning process. Health education cannot happen spontaneously; it requires a series of organised and directed educational influences, focused on the model of the person being formed. We begin by reviewing the historically significant progress in health education that has been shaken up during the recent pandemic caused by the SARS Cov 2 virus. After evidence emerged of the threat posed by these viruses, education accelerated the development of science to exponential stages in order to acquire the knowledge necessary to develop vaccines against them.

The training of health professionals, in its development, has largely preserved the provisions of the Flexner Report of 1910 and the Edinburgh II Declaration of 1993, creating the necessary conditions and guidelines for the optimal training of future professionals.

In the traditional flexnerist teaching model with positivist epistemology, undergraduate training in the health professions is characterised by a learning cycle with an emphasis on content where students learn various subjects within the basic sciences, and then develop the cycle of clinical topics from semiotics, combined with research concepts.

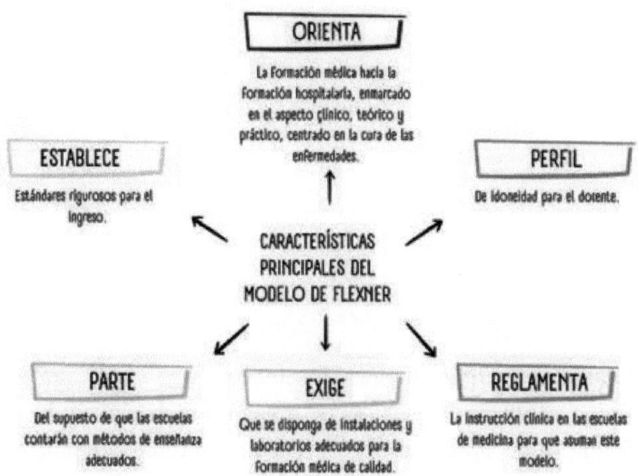

Figure 1. Main characteristics of the Flexnerian model

Innovations in current curricula are framed around providing greater flexibility, strengthening research competences, and virtuality. The adjective flexnerian was coined for medical training programmes with a clear division between the initial phase of the programme or core discipline, the second cycle dedicated to continuous research and skills development, and research; this model is widely used by most medical schools in Latin America. However, in the ever-changing world of education, where technology and innovation are ever protagonists, we are experiencing a renaissance of project-based learning, an approach that has the potential to change the way we think about learning, where students are active creators of the learning process and knowledge, not just its promoters. Thinking outside the box and finding creative solutions to problems that arise is part of the challenge of knowledge sharing.

Some researchers, with whom we fully agree, have analysed the current situation and concluded that, taking into account the change of practices in the health field, students should deepen their knowledge in humanities, administration, clinical epidemiology, exact sciences, information and communication technologies. The training methods should be extended from university and hospital classrooms to the local community.

Nowadays changes in science are advancing rapidly with trends and new health needs. This raises the possibility of contributing to the wider field of health, where knowledge must be integrated into culture, as over time what we call Homo Sapiens becomes what we believe. The above assumptions are part of the new challenges to be considered as developers of current health research programmes.

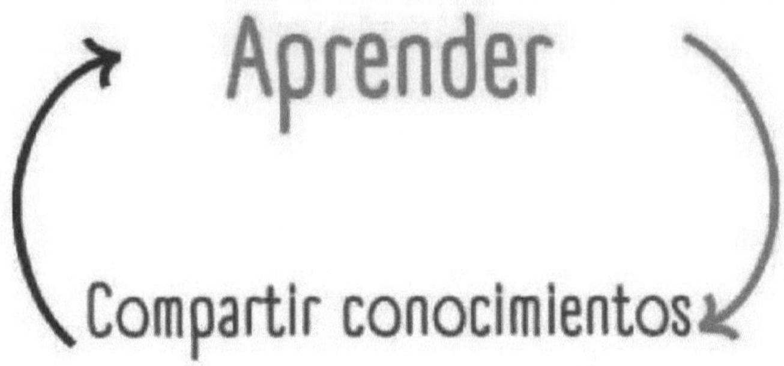

Figure 2. Learning cycle in the health sciences

The development of curricula with a greater emphasis on basic science laboratory studies, the strengthening of teaching-service agreements between health care institutions and universities, and the use of new technological communication tools have provided greater opportunities for the training of new health professionals.

Since Flexner presented his proposal until today, many changes in medical practice have led to the need to propose a comprehensive revision of training programmes for health professionals, focusing on the expected development of professionals in this new knowledge society.

The training programmes have embraced concepts of the researchers Jean Piaget and Lev. Semenovich Vygotsky; they suggest the development of new and innovative didactic strategies, all relevant to the professional context; students must be trained to analyse various situations around them, being able to implement feasible, practical, logical and concrete solutions. It is possible to consider the great influence in the field of health, which has been studied and analysed in depth by different authors in the course of the last decades.

Many researchers have underlined the great influence by stating that: Within the positivist universe of Flexnerianism there is a well-delineated equation that was reflected and shaped, which was imposed on the world over time: where the quality of training of health professionals is equal to the ability to master and correctly apply the principles that are held in the biological and clinical health disciplines. Undoubtedly, health education still revolves around Flexner's cognitive assumptions and any attempt to change the curricula implemented by academies starts with the recognition of his principles. A typical example is the offer of a course structure based not only on scientific disciplines, but also on major and important health topics, and even courses based on training in different settings. These proposals for curriculum development are clearly framed within the hegemony postulated by Flexner.

Some academic institutions have established professional training from undergraduate in the clinical cycle to postgraduate in medical and surgical specialities; using the Problem Based Learning method, in which a process of reflective analysis is developed by the student to provide solutions to each clinical case, which allows the development of clinical judgement as part of the professional competences (generic and specific) that will be extended every six months.

The pedagogical strategy based on problem solving as the educational model to follow, currently existing at both McMaster and Harvard, with the implementation of programmes to train tutors to be able to employ this strategy in a selection of documented cases. One of the arguments for this model is that it is able to guide clinical cases by integrating basic and clinical sciences. As with any new approach that seeks to change the way educational processes are understood, problem-based learning is seen as an appropriate step away from the old way of teaching knowledge from the teacher to the student.

New innovative models such as that of the Faculty of Medicine of the Autonomous University of Barcelona (UAB) has promoted the teaching of health sciences, with an integrated model that brings together the studies of medicine, health areas and physiotherapy in the same educational context.

Such has been the impact of the inclusion of information and communication technologies in the educational process that medical programmes and medical specialties have been established with curricula moving from face-to-face to virtual learning.

New York University has created a multidisciplinary curriculum where training is provided to future graduates in areas such as computer skills workshops, characterising computer resources, support in creating evidence-based research strategies, among other skills. The Medical University of South Carolina integrates computer science and computer technology learning into a compulsory course in the first semesters.

The training of health science professionals must result in a key, autonomous specialist qualification that demonstrates cross-cutting and specific professional competence in practice. By awarding the academic degree, the university certifies or recognises the competence of graduates, which must not endanger patients, society or any of its members.

Table 1. New subject proposal for medicine, nursing and physiotherapy

Medicine					
Course	**Sem.**	**Subject**	**Character**	**ECTS**	**Subject**
					Propaedeutic

1		Introduction to the health sciences	FB	6	of the sciences of the health
1		Cell biology	FB	6	Biology
Annual		Human Anatomy I	FB	9	Anatomy human
		Biophysics	FB	7	Physics
		Biostatistics	FB	6	Statistics
		Human biochemistry and molecular biology	FB	12	Biochemistry
2	1	Medical psychology	FB	6	Psychology
		Medical Physiology I	FB	8	Physiology
	2	Medical physiology II	FB	8	Physiology
	Annual	Microscopic structure of devices and systems	FB	6	Histology
		Human Anatomy II	FB	9	Human anatomy
		Total basic training		**83**	
Nursing					
1	1	Body structure human	FB	6	Anatomy human
		Psychosocial sciences	FB	6	Psychology
		Function of the human body I	FB	6	Physiology
		Scientific methodology and biostatistics	FB	6	Statistics
		Culture, society and health	FB	6	Sociology
	2	Communication and ICTs	FB	6	Communication
		Function of the human body II	FB	6	Physiology
		Nutrition	FB	6	Nutrition
		Total basic training		**66**	
Physiotherapy					
1	1	Human Anatomy I	FB	6	Human anatomy
		Biological basis of the human body	FB	9	Physiology

		Biophysics and biomechanics	FB	6	Biophysics
		Scientific methodology and biostatistics	FB	6	Statistics
		Function of the human body	FB	9	Physiology
	2	Human anatomy	FB	6	Human anatomy
		Human psychology	FB	6	Psychology
2	1	Clinical pathological concepts. Diagnostic techniques	FB	6	Human pathology
	2	Medico-surgical pathology	FB	6	Human pathology
		Total basic training		**60**	

Source: A multiprofessional learning model in health sciences: teaching innovation as a response to the emerging needs of our society.

Table 1 shows the basic training subjects of the three degrees. In italics are shown all those subjects that are likely to allow shared teaching, either totally or partially, among the various student profiles of the faculty, based on the availability of the teachers, the response given by the students themselves, the periodic evaluation and the results obtained in the learning process.
Knowledge sharing becomes an efficient pedagogical tool that facilitates the appropriate formulation of learning.

Human talent	Innovation Research	Renewed responsiveness in situations of collective health hazards
Integration of the social sector		

Figure 3. Intersectorality in Health

Figure 3 integrates the vision of interprofessional education to intervene in collective health from the concept of social determinants.
We cannot complete our understanding of the training of new health professionals without an assessment of local health systems. With the emergence of SARS Cov 2, international health has given way to global health, leading to a profound change of perspective. States and institutions can no longer see health as an issue bounded by national borders, as was the case in the past. Indeed, global health has become so important that it is of increasing

concern to civil society activists, as demonstrated by the clear impact on public policy and spending patterns in several countries.

The vast increase in contact across national borders, from travel to trade, has facilitated the spread of infectious diseases from one country to another and has created a broad and comprehensive understanding that infectious diseases can be spread from one country to another.

infectious diseases know no borders. On the other hand, the development of electronic communication has facilitated awareness of these changes.

Recent health threats, such as monkeypox, the Mòjiãng virus, the Langya virus, are global, and have contributed greatly to the awareness that health issues are now the concern of society, not just *health* workers.

Global health has indeed become everyone's concern: policy makers, funders, diplomats, a wide range of health service providers, activists, civil society groups, and citizens around the world.

Non-state actors have become increasingly necessary and the generation of global health partnerships has made them an important aspect at the international level. While these partnerships were created to make targeted health aid more effective, their overlapping and unclear mandates, as well as their tendency to be highly problem-focused, have made it difficult to channel donors to recipient countries and to manage foreign aid.

Most countries lack specific programmes; national research programmes that fund the best scientists. With visible leadership and buy-in for all major pandemic initiatives, we need to monitor their progress, test ideas, implement the most successful ones, and make sure they become products that can be rapidly developed. Without proper planning, when the next big outbreak occurs, governments will react, and it will be too late because we will have to try to plan while the pandemic is already spreading, which is not the right way to go about protecting the community.

Intervention strategies for public health outbreaks or incidents must be as clear and rigorous as the best military strategies in the world. The global healthcare landscape is increasingly driven by public-private partnerships. Thus, former UN Secretary General Kofi Annan launched the Global Health Initiative at the World Economic Forum in 2002 to engage business in public-private partnerships to fight HIV/AIDS, malaria, tuberculosis and improve health systems. The importance of foundations such as the Bill and Melinda Gates Foundation to global health makes it now one of the largest investors, having committed nearly $10 billion to global health aid. UNITAID an international mechanism for the procurement of drugs for the treatment of HIV/AIDS, tuberculosis and malaria. Many organisations are engaged in efforts that must be articulated and integrated to better respond to the growing challenges in global public health.

Of the national governments, we should highlight the efforts of the United States which formerly operated primarily through the United States Agency for International Development (USAID), but now there are a wide range of agencies that play an important role in global health: The National Institutes of Health, which sponsors research and development. Research opportunities; Centers for Disease Control and Prevention with health surveillance and technical cooperation programmes in many countries. The growing importance of health in US foreign policy is reflected in the creation of a special office of international health affairs in the State Department.

In the aftermath of the coronavirus pandemic, WHO's leadership is seen by many observers as ineffective and weak, despite its constitutional mandate to act as the guiding and coordinating authority for international health. Simultaneously, however, global programmes and public-private partnerships have become important in the overall commitment to global health.

The creation of a Global Epidemic Response and Mobilisation Team (GERM) linked to the WHO and staffed by 3,000 experts in epidemiology, data systems, genetics, medicines and even logistics is a social imperative to preserve the health of an increasingly interconnected planet. Containing a virus outbreak within 100 days of its appearance is the main challenge we face; we understand that outbreaks are not preventable, pandemics are. This with the help of a database that scientists and innovators have access to, in order to identify outbreaks, analyse the severity of the situation, take action and work on the study and production of tests, treatments and new vaccines.

This is why new advances in technologies and their implementation in almost all areas of training of health professionals in the world are an effective and indispensable tool for the proper development of the processes of generation and administration, making effective models of knowledge sharing, which develop timely interventions in individual and collective health.

With regard to the international and national vision on the challenges and opportunities of changing the care model and its relationship with the processes of organising interdisciplinary teams and the opening up of new scenarios (school-territories). It is clear that we are immersed in a dynamic process that seeks progress towards universal health with a focus on equity within a framework of rights.

The state as a health authority pursues greater social cohesion, which is necessary for better outcomes when it strengthens its governance capacities in essential public health functions by broadening the frontline of responsibilities

with national actors.
The model of care based on Primary Health Care with the organisation of teams with assigned territories and population is a basic principle for guaranteeing access to health.

Chapter 3

Training of Health Professionals: Challenges for Higher Education Institutions Facing

Higher Education Institutions Facing Integrated Care

Knowledge is not definitive; it is also possible to think that the university is not the centre of absolute knowledge.

Arnaldo Guédez

Health professionals inherently have multiple functions that comprise complex situations to be resolved, both with regard to the patient and their family, the organisation for which they work, the health professionals in the health care institutions, which is why, from their training, students demand to possess administrative knowledge for decision making that will enable them to direct actions in favour of the well-being of the user and the organisation when they are professionals. In general, experience has been configured in the work of health professionals, their work as the main factor in generating this type of knowledge, learning to treat patients, relatives and to perform within the different instances of interaction in health institutions.

Despite its relevance, one of the great challenges of health systems is the generation and continuity of the skills of health professionals, and to overcome this it is important that training programmes are in line with national and international trends, both in pedagogical aspects and in managerial and health knowledge of education processes as a way to provide solutions to the problems they face on a daily basis (Dandicourt, 2016); Therefore, it is considered relevant, necessary and pertinent to train and evaluate students in health areas based on the achievement of expected performances, reviewing their activities and results (Trincado and Fernández, 1995).

Thus, it is understood that the exercise of the health professional does not only imply the development of direct care, technical and instrumental activities, but also the implementation of various social, institutional and health functions, for which an amalgam of knowledge must be put into practice, applying the scientific method to practical problems in the reality of care. By virtue of this, the purpose of training is to prepare professionals with ethical principles, a humanistic perspective, a sense of social responsibility, knowledge, competences and skills to lead health services by applying management and leadership and, within this, management to lead care services involves planning, organisation, evaluation and control. For this reason, in addition to the disciplinary areas of humanities, research, basic sciences and management-administrative knowledge should be included in the curricula of the degree programme as essential knowledge in the new times (Barbera et al., 2015).

Barbera et al. (2015) show that scientific evolution, the increase in the demands of users and the increase in patient care lead them to consider it essential for the practice of health professionals that educational institutions can generate proposals that link both theoretical models and practical activities. Thus, from the perspective of the authors, it will be possible to develop the skills and competencies required for positions in this area. Therefore, a line of relationship must be established between the technical and personal skills, the capacities and the learning outcomes of health professionals in the administrative/managerial area.

It should be noted that, worldwide, health professionals such as doctors, nurses, physiotherapists, nutritionists and others have been affected by legislative changes, which have a direct impact on the competences and profiles that this profession should have. In Europe, for example, legislative proposals for the convergence of curricula have been studied, increasingly involving critical thinking as an important competence. Underpinning these revisions is the consideration that care for health professionals must be based on competences aimed at efficiency (Clavijo et al., 2016).

In addition to this, Bautista-Espinel et al. (2017) highlight that the practice of health areas demands a distinctive pattern of knowledge within the health team. And these patterns, or models, are necessary for professional discernment and expertise, which must be enunciated, and learnt, in an integral way in order to manage the interventions of the case. Thus, it is necessary to know how to coordinate, plan, organise and execute actions in an interdisciplinary way in order to lead and manage the care of people.

Thus, the education of health professionals, for example in the areas of health, must be based on excellence and leadership. In this sense Guerrero-Núñez and Cid-Henríquez (2015) consider that this process is perceived as an action that is oriented to direct, manage, and develop activities to control in different areas of the usual actions, taking into account the characteristics that determine them; notable step for obtaining answers from the hospital scenario, contextualising the emergency in support of the management of services in critical situation.

It should be noted that the practice of health students can strengthen the theoretical knowledge , managing that the autonomous advancement of the work manifests the growth and consolidation of the legal capacity to support the work of the professional. These skills come from the actions generated by the management, execution, diagnosis and medical treatment of health areas, guaranteeing that patients receive the best management of aid resources.

In addition, it is the opinion of Betancourt-Gonzales (2020) that universities with health programmes, especially, must guarantee comprehensive training in which professionals can use knowledge to make decisions about patient care, take into account patient preferences and values, and incorporate experience into their work.

For the authors, as for Soto-Fuentes et al. (2014), in order to obtain an appropriate practice of integrated work in health professionals, students must broaden their interpersonal skills during university training, which will allow them to work in an interdisciplinary manner to provide the best comprehensive care to people in health services. Thus, the aim is to provide students with practice scenarios that allow interaction and assertive communication in order to propose efficient solutions to the problems presented.

Therefore, new educational trends require the incorporation, from the curriculum, of competences that develop professionalism. The aim is for them to be able to face changes in organisations in order to respond to the demands of patients, strengthening their skills and abilities, maintaining suitable and effective communication and basing the management of the process on regulations, but also on the ethical principles of comprehensive care (Bustamante García, 2021).

It is validly stated that the training characteristics of professionals play an important role in determining competences and job performance. For this reason, it is necessary to move from the training processes of disintegrated, disjointed and/or fragmented knowledge in the curricular spaces to the development of soft and hard skills and abilities in communication, conflict resolution and leadership (Soto-Fuentes et al., 2014), typologies that are necessary for adequate administrative management in the health services. The curricular content of health programmes should comprehensively address all those elements required for the training of these professionals, with a view to seeking coordinated results in terms of the content of the subject. This should contribute to the benefit of the programmes, generating new knowledge, in such a way that it can be aligned with some of the learning outcomes expected after graduation.

The academy has a high social responsibility to train health professionals from a holistic point of view, so that they can respond to all administrative management needs in health care institutions.

According to Valenzuela (2016), in the service or professional practice spaces, students can, and should, have the possibility, individually or in groups, to characterise, inspect and consider the patient within an environment in which care actions converge, promoting improvements in the health condition of those they attend. At the same time, it must be assumed that globalisation has brought about changes in different contexts with regard to the development of health care, such as: the existence of problems in the world economy, the rise of technology, the conception and responsibilities of the State, a deep-rooted difference between public and private scenarios, and the prevalence of high competition between economic and social sectors to be favoured with the management of economic resources (Feo, 2003). Another aspect of relevance is the demands of patients on health caregivers, requiring competent professionals, with skills and abilities, decisive, leaders in the management of care, processes of change and policy reforms for the welfare of public health, as well as their profession (Paravic, 2010).

In principle, academic programmes for the training of health professionals must ensure that the training of these professionals is supported by high competencies that they can provide in health care. This must be underpinned by the management of planning, organising processes, generating motivation plans for trainees, as well as establishing controls that activate protocols for the provision of adequate, safe and comprehensive care and attention. This is to ensure that the care provided is as expected. In this context, the process of care supported by strategies aligned to the achievement of benefit, such as quality health care, must be taken into account (De Arco-Canoles & Suárez-Calle, 2018).

According to Milos et al. (2010) and Ceballos-Vásquez et al. (2015) in this case, they refer to the training of nurses, who have management responsibility, not only in the economic resources of the services they lead, but also in reference to the human and structural aspect. The latter aspect is oriented towards providing excellent care, acquiring legal responsibilities. This implies assuming expert autonomy, as a determined and different action from other professions in the health area, for which there are functions that are only their responsibility, being non-delegable. In this context, professional discernment is required, developed with and for a planned context that involves different tasks aligned with the fulfilment of objectives, i.e. their execution. This must respond to the needs of planning, organising and executing interdisciplinary work to achieve comprehensive health care, within the health team, they are responsible for leading the process and ensuring the proper management of resources and supplies for patient care.

Therefore, Higher Education Institutions (HEIs) must ensure that students of health professions acquire training competences from different approaches, in order to have a professional who knows, anticipates and promotes the new trends in health care: updating knowledge and practice, globally, leading professionals in health services, who are the guarantor of all resources, both economic and others that facilitate comprehensive care, who ensure the good management of resources that give sustainability to the health system. And in this, González- Esteban et al. (2016) highlight that creating motivational relationships is essential.

In the opinion of Pat et al. (2021), there are several studies that indicate that the training of human resources in health requires moving away from rigid and hierarchical models, in favour of new leadership structures, which are conceived as malleable and open, allowing for the opening of combined spaces for discernment. In this aspect, the health professional appropriates knowledge from science, occupying a place in the context of the general health method. Thus, it is relevant for organisations to teach professionals about leadership strategies, auditing, decision-making, resource management, among other administrative-managerial aspects that distinguish them in the management of health service organisations.

In the opinion of Latrach-Anmar et al. (2011), education in administrative-managerial competencies during theoretical-practical training is a central element in the improvement of health professionals, and is considered a key factor in guaranteeing the quality of work and personal quality of those who will be responding to the shortcomings of comprehensive health care. In this sense, capacity and good professional practice are directly associated with theoretical knowledge, together with discernment, analysis and clinical reasoning, in order to be able to strengthen skills and take actions that facilitate problem solving. In short, evaluation is associated with the generation of skills that permeate towards the linking of interpersonal relationships, interceding in the management administrative management.

The concept of competence for the training of human talent in health incorporates the learning of knowledge and procedural skills, as well as all those aspects of the professional being linked to behavioural skills, interpersonal relationships, teamwork and reflective critical thinking. These must be verified in the professional profile in order to work efficiently, with the ability to adapt quickly and effectively to emerging changes, face uncertainty and make decisions in accordance with the context in which it corresponds to act (Garavito, 2019).

The set of administrative actions that health care trainees have to face in order to manage care requires hierarchical authority and autonomy, technological, economic and regulatory knowledge, which can only be acquired through knowledge and practice. This occurs because they are moralistic conflicts confronted by professionals in their experience, which arise from work action. Thus, the focus of comprehensive care is deepened in the essence that sustains this profession, which is relevant in the new and precipitated administrative tendencies, by virtue of the labour plots that the scenarios attribute to health professionals. From this we can see the need to obtain administrative knowledge to direct and manage care, focusing on quality control processes, associated with efficiency and productivity. All of the above must be established taking into account the control mechanisms and monitoring actions on the financial process, coexisting as a necessary action rooted in the new global care trends, which have to be faced in the health system (Gaviria, 2009). Hence the importance of training these health professionals in competencies in administrative-managerial knowledge with a theoretical-practical approach during training. This will allow the student to acquire administrative competencies, achieving an exhaustive learning of the actions carried out, demonstrating their successes and opportunities in decision-making, leadership, initiative and assertive problem-solving skills in relation to all the activities they have to carry out in the context of the administrative area in the different health care institutions where they carry out their internships.

According to Gómez (2013), education in administrative and managerial competences for students in health training programmes allows them to integrate the theoretical knowledge imparted in the classroom with the numerous examples that can be identified in the action of the process itself ( ). This favours professional alignment with integrity, competence and morality, which is why it is necessary to have suitable environments that are normatively approved by the biosafety conditions defined for this purpose.

Therefore, the professions in training for health care (doctors, nurses, physiotherapists, nutritionists, etc.), it is the academy that must ensure the teaching and evaluation of the learning of administrative and managerial competences in order to demonstrate real learning in this area of training, taking into account the need of the system and organisations (Pérez et al., 2017).

Continuing to train professionals under traditional curricula is a short-sighted vision that does not see the processes of training and assessment of administrative competences as a felt need that reflects the new trends of holistic professionals, who master the administrative and managerial contexts to provide care to users in health organisations, This should be seen not only as isolated learning in the curricula, but as a form of integral learning for professionals, fulfilling an accrediting function of the administrative teaching process integrated into the management of each process required in the services for user care, whether at the hospital or outpatient level.

In contrast to this, teaching and evaluation processes have to be related to the

management of objectives linked to the administrative elements of decision-making, which, in addition, must be approached in a rational and effective way, given that, as an ongoing activity within professional practice, they require a holistic and comprehensive vision, especially in processes used by health programmes (Kruger et al. 2017).
Based on these considerations, Chaves et al. (2010) propose in a study the creation of the *Developing a Curriculum* (DACUM) method, which encompasses different strategies from the various contexts of action of health professionals for curriculum development.
This method of Canadian origin is designed with a standard language that assimilates requirements of knowledge, aptitudes, concrete and universal skills, expertise and forms required for a specific position or set of actions in the workplace. For this reason, this technique is used by several governments and organisations to represent functions and competencies of positions, occupations or to deploy study plans that are used to help train human talent, for career projection, classification of people, execution of aptitude models, preparation and development of courses.
This is achieved by incorporating competency-based training. In this regard, the Ministry of Health (2018) states that:
The competency-based approach guides the training and management processes of human talent in the area of health, in order to provide relevant and comprehensive responses to the health needs of the population, within the framework of the health system, integrating the knowledge, skills, attitudes and qualities that must be present in human talent for the proper exercise of their professions and occupations. This perspective implies that the training processes that take place inside and outside educational institutions should be permanently fed back to the context in which the human talent works or will work, strengthening the link between academia, health services and the population and promoting new forms of evaluation and performance measurement systems (p.49). (p.49).
In addition, the National Academy of Medicine and the Ministry of Health and Social Protection (2013) show that the General Social Security System - which emerged from Law 100 of 1993, together with the reforms of Law 1122 of 2009 and Law 1438 of 2011 - has been shaping the occupational profile of health experts. Among them, the profile of health professionals stands out especially, due to the progressive delegation of occupations of an administrative nature, with the constant reduction of time and appropriate environments to devote to their professional role. And, in the midst of this, the need to improve the training of health professionals is established.

In this regard, the Ministry of Health (2018) states that:
More decisive health teams are required to address the main problems and epidemiological characteristics of the Colombian population. This implies considering the restrictions that the health system has to meet the growing demand for specialised services, due to high costs and the unavailability of sufficient specialists to meet a demand for this type of service similar to that of more developed countries in the medium term. The health and education systems must focus on the development of adequate competencies in the human talent available in the country and its regions, in order to achieve their objectives. The competencies approach guides the processes of training and management of human talent in the area of health, in order to provide relevant and comprehensive responses to the health needs of the population, within the framework of the health system, integrating the knowledge, skills, attitudes and qualities that should be present in human talent for the proper exercise of their professions and occupations. . This perspective implies that the training processes that take place inside and outside educational institutions must be permanently fed back to the context in which the human talent works or will work, strengthening the link between academia, health services and the population and promoting new forms of evaluation and performance measurement systems. (p. 49)
Thus, from the national regulations it is considered necessary to think about the quality and relevance of the training of health professionals, with those of health areas, as a result of the development of capacities that show soft skills for interpersonal relations, adaptation and leadership. Now, this recognition seems to be a response to the fact that the reform of the Health System, arising from Law 100 of 1993, was carried out without prior studies on the changes that it would bring to the human talent in health and what its impact would be on the IPS and educational institutions to train the new professionals required by the system. The above ratifies the commitment that health professionals must have to develop actions aimed at complying with all the requirements of the health sector, in which they play an important role, as they are responsible for leading and managing care services at any level of care.
Health professionals provide leadership on crucial health issues, proportion the research agenda and stimulate the production, transfer and dissemination of valuable knowledge. Therefore, higher education institutions should establish and promote the participation of health areas in different areas in addition to public health, these health professionals acquire the expert knowledge base, capable of making complex decisions during their work, with clinical competencies for a broad practice, whose characteristics are determined by the

context and/or the country in which they work. During their training, health professionals must become qualified to opt for a comprehensive research, educational, clinical and management practice, obtain a high level of professional autonomy and independence in practice, develop decision-making skills and diagnostic logic.

Similarly, educational institutions in Colombia have undertaken new training searches that are in tune with the professional and labour trends required by healthcare systems. In view of this, Morfi (2010) describes that Care Management:

As in the case of health professionals, it is defined as the application of professional judgement in planning, organising, motivating and controlling the provision of timely, safe, comprehensive care that ensures continuity of care and is based on strategic guidelines, in order to obtain health as the final product. (p.1)

In turn, authors such as Soto-Fuentes et al. (2014) state that:

The training of health professionals, including health professionals as process leaders, plays a fundamental role in the composition and dynamics of the workforce, in the quality and relevance of care, and in the development of institutional capacity in health. Therefore, they demonstrate competence when they effectively apply a combination of knowledge, skills and clinical judgement in daily practice or job performance (p.82).

In this sense, health methods all over the world are investigating strategies, structures and ways of working in a better cost-effective way, in order to provide the best care to users and their families, based on current scientific evidence. Therefore, Soto-Fuentes et al. (2014) argue that the learning of health professionals is transformative and implies deploying leadership conditions, with the intention of constituting professionals who stand out as agents of change. This ability must mobilise both academic communities and experts and is a crucial factor for the success of reform efforts in academic institutions.

Bearing all of the above in mind, Colombia urgently requires the implementation of more decisive health teams to carry out the care of problems. It is worth mentioning that the health system is being constrained by the demand for specialised services for reasons such as high costs and the unavailability of efficient specialists to provide quality care.

Consequently, health and education systems must implement appropriate strategies to develop more than cognitive and theoretical competencies, those related to human talent and the fulfilment of objectives. In other words, a competency-based approach should be carried out, oriented towards training and management processes of human talent in the health area that allows for the recognition of irregularities and/or health needs of the population (Ministry of Health, 2018).

Also, if it is considered that health professionals also cover disease prevention and health promotion, as well as user care, and the interpersonal relationships that result from this, administrative-managerial issues are outside the scope of what is expected of them. In this case, administrative management is understood as the set of coordinated tasks and activities that help to make optimal use of the resources an organisation possesses, making decisions on allocation and distribution of resources, in order to achieve the objectives and obtain the best results. In this aspect, interdisciplinarity is relevant, allowing the student to acquire the necessary knowledge to carry out his or her function as a professional.

Thus, both the most recent legislation and the different doctrinal articles and literature on the subject coincide in pointing out the necessary complementarity between the training of health professionals and the administrative and managerial experience of these professionals, as well as the balance between theory and practice in order to achieve a complete and comprehensive work.

Therefore, this aspect is important and relevant, since students who are being trained in health professions must have administrative/managerial competences, which are becoming increasingly important in the management of health services in order to provide comprehensive care, guarantee resources for care and manage leadership that focuses on managing, auditing and directing care processes in order to guarantee quality care.

The education of health professionals is focused on providing comprehensive care, therefore, it must be addressed holistically, and for this, training is required that favours the interaction of knowledge to plan health care. Thus, the elements required to update knowledge must be established in theoretical knowledge in order to give pedagogical support to practice. It is hoped that the learning during the theoretical and practical development will allow the acquired knowledge to make sense as an essential ingredient in the meaningful experience. The processes taught must be interesting and must allow the interaction of previous and new concepts, in such a way that they contribute to modifying, changing and structuring curricula and, therefore, re-evaluating comprehensive care in the new work contexts is undoubtedly a responsibility of higher education institutions, with regard to the training of health professionals and the new training and work trends to face the new challenges of demands and health care (Morfi, 2010).

This also supports the root cause that more and more administrative responsibilities are delegated to health professionals. Therefore, Higher Education Institutions (HEIs) that train these professionals must re-evaluate the competencies of students in this area of knowledge, in order to be increasingly competent, according to the new labour trends required by health organisations in the face of the challenges and labour competitiveness, based on financial sustainability (Guerrero-Núñez and Cid-Henríquez, 2015).

Chapter 4

Towards a New Model

We can't be in survival mode. We have to be in growth mode Jeff Bezos

Integrated Health Management is a concept that has penetrated with force in the panorama of health care institutions worldwide, especially thanks to the innovation that New Technologies are experiencing and their impact on the development of the so-called Information Society. The concept of integrated health management is not homogeneous. However, all authors emphasise the importance of coordinating the provision of high quality services under specific conditions, using the appropriate resources given the technical-scientific circumstances, in order to achieve the best results. The health system, then, must be understood as something broader than the health care system, which has as its social components civil society and the market, the non-state public sector and the state itself, where public health covers a part of the care system in the private sector, in the non-state public sector and in the state sector.

After the pandemic scenario, we are obliged not only to be prepared to face new diseases, but also to prevent possible future needs that may arise before the occurrence of outbreaks or cases, and to achieve this we must maintain an active epidemiological surveillance, implementing a culture of creativity that allows us to be at the forefront to make the necessary changes before these events become social crises in health. According to the formulation of the essential public health function No. 5, institutional capacity for public health management is defined by five components: leadership and communication, evidence-based decision making, strategic planning, organisational development and resource management, especially human and financial.

In Colombia, despite the advances in health, the serious problems facing the sector have not been resolved: the dominant role of the Health Promoting Companies (EPS), the fragmentation and disintegration of care; low resolution capacity; vertical integration, high disease burden; market failures; negative incentives among agents and regulatory failure, which has led to increased inequity; in a health service delivery model focused mainly on morbidity and centred on actors; dehumanised; decontextualised and without prevalence of rights. The doctor-patient relationship has been seriously affected, as well as the weighting of health professionals in the exercise of their medical act, often questioned or stigmatised without scientific basis.

With the enactment of Resolution 429 of 2016, the aim was to generate better conditions for the population through the regulation of sectoral and intersectoral intervention, which seeks to strengthen Primary Health Care.

Retaking the Primary Care model with a family and community approach, care and comprehensive risk management and the differential approach, aims to achieve the articulation and harmonisation of the provision of health services and the development of public health policies and programmes through social management processes and intersectoral policy.
On the other hand, integrated health management seeks to strengthen healthy lifestyles in communities, based on the promotion of a culture of self-care through communication campaigns and specific programmes. An analysis of health situations is carried out, in accordance with the determinants established in Mark Lalonde's model.
Integrated management is moving towards a Primary Health Care strategy, with a family and community focus, to guarantee timeliness, continuity, accessibility, comprehensiveness and quality. One of the challenges in Primary Health Care actions is the training of professionals with specific knowledge and skills for the implementation of the strategy and with a socio-cultural approach.

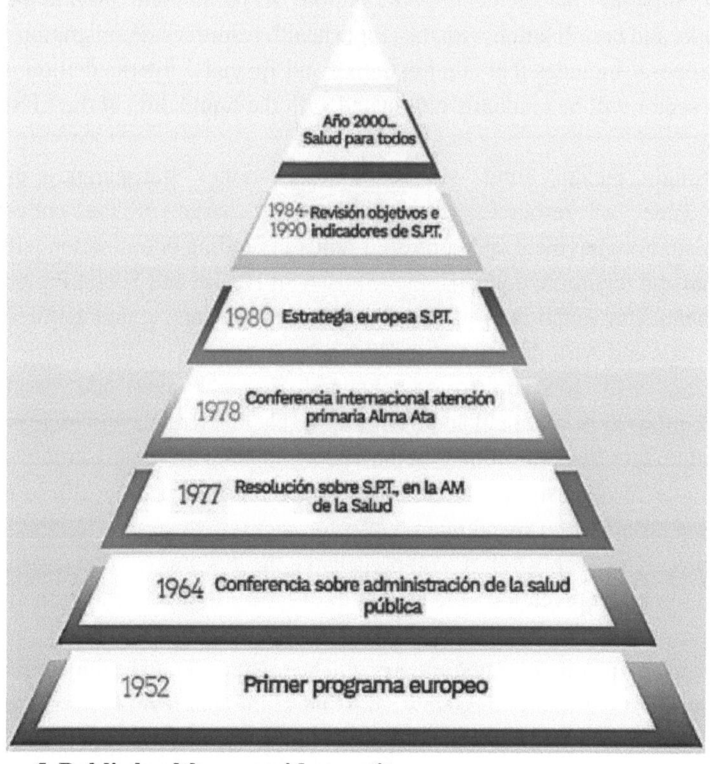

Figure 5. Public health pyramid over time

The role of health professionals is to provide education, prevent illness and ensure the necessary quality and availability of care. In addition, there are other transversal (or non-specific) competences equally necessary for good professional practice based on the interpersonal aspects of care, in terms of the ability to perceive the needs and understand the disease situations in which patients find themselves. Developing conceptual and analytical thinking; maintaining a high level of self-confidence, excellent interpersonal skills and the ability to work in a team.

In the current context we must refer to the Government Programme for an era of peace announced by the elected president of Colombia, which is framed by the following proposals in the area of health:

Democratic and participatory governance: a single public health system, governed by a National Health Council and with territorial councils that will include indigenous and Afro-descendant people. The councils will be made up of health authorities and delegates from communities, workers, scientific societies, the private sector and academia. Their functions are to direct health policy, integral management, coordination of public and private benefit networks and coordination with the single health resource administration fund. The proposal includes that administrative and financial intermediation in the health sector will be gradually eliminated with the liquidation of the EPSs and ARLs.

The Single Health Fund will serve to guarantee transparency in the management of resources, and will be in charge of the collection, administration, payment and control of funds in binding coordination with the national and territorial councils, the Ministry of Health and Social Protection, and the health authorities at the level of departments, municipalities and indigenous and Afro-descendant territories.

Financing will continue to be obtained through taxes and parafiscal contributions at the national and territorial levels in a tendency to increase the general budget by controlling evasion and avoidance, increasing employment and labour formalisation, and aiming for public spending on health to be no less than 80% of total spending in the sector.

The proposal establishes a comprehensive health model that prioritises promotion and prevention, and will improve care and rehabilitation with a human rights, intercultural and differential approach (Agora, 2022).

According to the proposal, the country will be organised into healthy territories for good living at the village, township and municipal levels. In rural areas: Specialised teams in different health areas will be organised to provide services and care in all areas. These teams will go directly to families in their homes, to

children in kindergartens and schools, to young people in universities and to workers and employers in workplaces where actions to prevent accidents and deaths at work will be intensified.
They are proposed as axes of public health policy, as described in Agora (2022):
-Achieve comprehensive care for pregnant women and early childhood, as well as comprehensive and universal neonatal screening.
-Achieve the goal of zero deaths from hunger, as well as fight overweight and obesity, tax sugary drinks, promote a healthy food industry.
-Dignified and comprehensive care for victims who suffered during the armed conflict.
-Reduce pollution and improve the quality of water, air and food; greater control over the use of toxic substances such as asbestos, mercury, lead and others.
Prevention and comprehensive care of hallucinogenic drug use with harm reduction approach through strategies such as mobile drug care centres.
Health services at the national level will be provided by a public-private network: Primary care will be provided by public hospitals in the framework of their territorial jurisdiction throughout the country with a focus on primary care and preventive health, population-based, resolutive, participatory and with high technological support. Medium and high complexity health services will be provided by public and private hospitals.
-Public spending will finance, without access barriers, benefits not excluded by law: the services covered by public financing will be all those that are not excluded as benefits according to the criteria of the Statutory Law 1751 and therefore there will be no administrative restrictions for any group of health technologies that have not been excluded.
-Health training for all levels and areas will be strengthened to achieve international level coverage indicators in the number of general practitioners, medical specialties, health areas and dentistry, among others, both in terms of averages and equitable distribution throughout the territory.
On the issue of medicines, achieving universal access at a fair cost to the country: these will be strengthened through price regulation and control, the declaration of public interest for the issuing of compulsory licences, public promotion of research and development of medicines, rational use based on cost-effectiveness analysis, good practices, strict pharmacovigilance and also through the availability of information.
This proposal aims to ensure the rationality of spending, strengthening all existing mechanisms to improve quality, timeliness, medical autonomy,

satisfaction, comprehensiveness, scientific validity and positive cost-benefit ratios.

To this end, it is necessary to clarify that these proposals must pass through the filter of the interests of the different actors in the sector, with the elimination of intermediation being of paramount importance, although this is perhaps the breaking point or the most critical point thanks to the great power of influence that the EPS unions currently have.

However, these points in some way propose viable alternatives and strategies to improve the system or any other health model. I hope that the reflections presented here are not only part of a text to be read again when an event of public health interest arises, so I invite you to continue reviewing the postulates that can easily be enriched with your comments and annotations; contributing from the academy to achieve a health system that improves in quality without affecting coverage, dignifying the health worker with fair and equitable salaries.

Chapter 5

Model for the Development of Health Management Systems

You will never change your life until you change something you do every day.
JOHN MAXWELL

The concept of quality management in health is developed through motivational, socially and culturally accepted models that can improve the determinants of the health of the population. Actions based on coercion or simple information processes that cannot affect the community are excluded from this concept. One of the pillars of social health in culture, Cliffdej J. Gertz defined it as a system of symbols. People communicated constantly through the system and established them throughout their lives. Bernardo Klicksberg defined it as a set of values of different groups; furthermore, he argued that culture is a determining factor for social cohesion. Unfortunately, many in our environment see culture as a secondary need to be addressed after other needs are considered a priority.

The taxonomy of the PLECOSER model succeeds in integrating positive points into a logical and simple process for planning and implementing activities to ensure high quality health care. The system is presented in an easily replicable process for improving the quality of health services. The quality of care provided by a health institution to its users is perceived through the characteristics of the care process; interpersonal relationships, consultation content, duration, clinical examination activities and diagnostics, improving health through physical, human and organisational attributes, which are central to the model.

The PLECOSER model is based on five main axes, namely:

1. Planning
2. Execution
3. Control
4. Follow-up
5. Feedback

PLANNING

It is the process and result of organising a simple or complex task, taking into account the composition of internal or external factors in order to achieve one or more objectives. Health management planning is key to achieving the desired results; in an organisation, it becomes the first step in achieving the institutional mission and vision. At the heart of the planning process is the ability to monitor current actions aimed at achieving desired objectives and to predict their future consequences.

Planning is a fundamental stage in decision-making that allows the ideal path to be traced in order to achieve organisational objectives. It takes into account internal and external factors that may influence the achievement of the established goals, elements of the current situation and values that will guide the organisation in its productive activities. Planning is a critical stage in the development of any project, as it lays the foundations and develops the necessary strategies. This is the basis of the project: identifying its essential elements, such as procedures, values, goals, etc., which form the framework for the organisation's activities. Careful planning is not necessarily a guarantee of success, but it is a solid starting point for anticipating problems and avoiding excessive improvisation with all the risks that this entails.

Statutory Law 1751 of 2015 expressly establishes that health is a fundamental autonomous right and in Article 12 of the same law, it states that "the fundamental right to health includes the right of people to participate in the decisions adopted by the agents of the health system that affect or interest them" and defines the scope of participation of the actors to actively participate in the formulation of health policy as well as in the plans to be implemented, and to participate in the promotion and prevention programmes that are established.

The Ministry of Health and Social Protection through Resolution 1536 of 2015 establishes the provisions for the process of Integrated Planning for Health in charge of territorial entities.

Resolution 1536 also includes the obligations of the Benefit Plan Administration Entities (EAPB) and the Labour Risks Administrators (ARL) to comply with the planning process by accepting and integrating the inputs that allow its execution. Chapter II of this Resolution defines the characterisation of the population that will be under the responsibility of the EAPBs and ARLs contemplated in the Benefit Plan; who must identify risks, prioritise populations within the affiliated persons and places within the territory, in order to prevent the individual interventions necessary to mitigate risks.

An effective and efficient process must be carried out:

1. Establish a quality policy, objectives of the health service provider institution, define the strategies to be socialised, trained and implemented at the different levels of care.

The company's quality policy is the written statement of the general management's commitment; its function is to:

- Communicate to the organisation that there is a decision to maintain the effort to meet the quality objectives.
- Establish that user needs and compliance with requirements are a

priority in the development of operational and administrative activities.

• It must be understood by all levels of the organisation, so that the activities to be carried out are done with this framework as a reference.

To this end, the following characteristics must be established:

• Recognise the raison d'être of the company: to seek to satisfy the requirements of users, both internal and external.

• Implement a process of continuous improvement, as requirements change over time and must be adapted to the market in order to be more competitive.

• Being the fundamental pillar for the company's performance, as it establishes the strategic definition of the company for a long period of work.

• Raise awareness among staff that the future of the company depends on the quality of the services provided.

• The quality policy designed should be dynamic and simply described so that it can be understood by all.

2. Quality management is directly related to productivity; quality management allows better results to be achieved with the same resources.

3. The need to establish the levels of responsibility and authority in the organisation, defining them in documents that record the authority, responsibility and operational and administrative relationships that are necessary to manage, execute and control the activities in order for this to be done with quality.

4. Leadership in the institution should be encouraged to provide solutions, follow up and implement planned actions to improve quality.

In order to comply with the concepts of responsibility and authority, it is necessary to clearly define each of the positions established.

The following elements must be taken into account as a minimum for the definition of the positions:

• Functional area: Describes the post to be defined.

• Objective: State the overall objective of the position.

• Duties: Describes the different activities to be performed in the job. It is made up of the following conditions:

- Definition of the activity carried out in the post, trying to present the most important activities.

- Objective of the activity. The particular objective of that particular action should be stated.

- Measurement. Establish mechanisms to measure the objectives of each activity; as indicators, these should preferably be statistical tools.

- Co-responsibility. Responsibilities are not exclusive, the achievement of objectives depends on teamwork, so co-responsibility must be determined; the person directly responsible for the activity is the person occupying the job that is being defined.

- It requires the identification and availability of the necessary resources to ensure the quality of products and services.
- There should be a clearly identified person within the institution responsible for the implementation of the quality assurance system, who should have a direct line to management to ensure that the system is established, implemented and maintained, and with a duty to report to management.
- Management should implement a control system, having as a tool for monitoring:

> Self-audits. As feedback on the state of the system, it is necessary to carry out self-audits in order to know the situation and compare it with the objectives and the established strategy.

> Committees. One of the most effective ways of assertively communicating and defining alternatives is through committees.

IMPLEMENTATION

This word, as such, comes from the Latin *exsecutio, exsecutiõnis.* In this sense, execution can be defined as to carry out or elaborate something, to perform an action or task, or to make something work. From an epistemological point of view, the project consists of 3 components that determine its origin and basic purpose. These components are: intention, information and decision-making. From a pragmatic point of view, project implementation refers to the execution of all the tasks foreseen in the project plan. You might think that the execution phase is the easiest of all phases, especially if you have already done the hardest part (planning) and laid the groundwork for the success of the project. But it is in the execution phase that many teams run into problems. When you start, organise all the tasks needed to achieve each objective: key human resources, capital requirements and budget. Identify any risk factors and consider measures to reduce risk. Review references to other required documents, such as required trainings.

In the framework of the PLECOSER model, this should include:

1. The IPS quality committee should be appointed and this group will assign specific responsibilities as planned and schedule budget expenditures for the smooth running of the system.

The procedure for institutional training will be established by the quality committee and reviewed periodically according to the schedule; at the end of each meeting minutes will be taken including discussions, conclusions, recommendations and summary of tasks.

Table 2. Quality committee responsibility matrix

Requirement	Area of the Company	Respon sable
1. Management responsibility		
2. Quality System		
3. Revision of the Contract		
4. Document and Data Control		
5. Procurement		
6. Control of Products Delivered by the Customer		
7. Identification and Traceability		
8. Process Control		
9. Inspection and Testing		
10. Control Inspection and Test Equipment		
11. Inspection and Test Status		
12. Control of non-conforming product		

13. Corrective and preventive actions		
14. Handling, storage, preservation and delivery		
15. Control of quality records		
16. Quality audits		
17. Training		
18. Service		
Statistical techniques		

Area Manager

Notes:

2. Awareness raising. All the organisation's staff must be aware of the project, its importance and the strategies that are being implemented in the process of implementing the quality assurance system.

Any change offers resistance, so a strong process of top management commitment and a strong socialisation and motivation of all staff is needed.

3. Training programme. IPSs must implement a comprehensive training programme for all staff according to a schedule presented in advance to all those involved.

The training programme is an important part of the implementation of the system, identifying methods, tools and ways of realising the system.

4. Development of the quality manual. The documentation of the quality management system is an essential part of achieving the expected results.

The preparation of the quality manual is one of the crucial steps, especially when there are management protocols, care guidelines, process and procedure manuals, formats, records, and these need to be changed according to the system being implemented.

In order to comply with the quality manual, the following sections are required:

- Define the organisation's quality policy.
- Design the organisation chart of the company, where responsibility and authority are established, resources and personnel for verification are indicated, and it is explicitly stated who is the person acting as the leader for the implementation of the quality system. The part corresponding to the responsibility, authority and other characteristics established in this point can be done by means of job descriptions in which the requirements of the standard are defined.
- Have contact with the user to clarify doubts or to ensure that they are on the appropriate route and compatible with the supplier's quality system; should be achieved through a representative, who makes reference to the person who will be the contact and responsible for following up to comply with

the standard, establishing their general data, position in the organisation to which they belong and how to contact them for any doubts, so that they comply with what is specified with their suppliers according to the product and the inspection and testing conditions that must be fulfilled.

- Establish the vital functions of each of the positions that are important for the control of the products and/or services being provided.
- Establish the company's general policies for action in relation to each of the requirements of the standard, in a way that allows others involved in the process to define their own systems and procedures.
- A list of the procedures that are applicable to the company for each of the requirements is integrated.
- As in all documents related to the standard, it is required to have a section for authorisations, revisions and control of the quality assurance manual.

CONTROL

Control is the main mechanism of the PLECOSER model, whose objective is to verify whether the protocols and objectives of the health institutions (IPS) comply with the established rules and regulations. Control is the stage of the management process that establishes standards to evaluate the results achieved in order to prevent deviations and continuously improve operations. The main function of controls is to prevent irregularities and correct factors that reduce the productivity and efficiency of the system.

It is a mechanism to avoid deviations in expected results within the organisational system that depends on the performance of the first two stages, especially the Planning stage. In theory, health institutions whose processes and results are closer to the plan will be more effective than those that deviate. Therefore, the monitoring process not only measures the performance of the organisation, but also determines the exact ideal quality standards for it, evaluates and takes related corrective actions.

In this sense, the ideal control process in health institutions should be economical, flexible and preventive, and, as we have said, it should include two fundamental elements: internal auditing and the measurement of user satisfaction.

- Internal audit. The internal health audit is considered a management control tool , because when this activity is carried out deliberately and in accordance with existing regulations, it creates a kind of mental map that shows the current state of the organisation and orients health personnel to take corrective action when necessary and to be at the forefront of improving and expanding the quality of health services.

• Measuring Satisfaction. By conducting user satisfaction surveys, it is possible to find out the extent to which user expectations are being met. Satisfaction surveys are closely related to strategies for maintaining and improving the quality of products and services. They are the starting point for decision making based on qualitative and quantitative information obtained from customer questionnaires.

FOLLOW-UP

After obtaining the initial data in the project, it is necessary to identify deviations and evaluate them in order to take actions to achieve the desired results. Monitoring is a resource that facilitates detailed observation of the operation and tests performed in order to make the right decisions at the right time. Each phase, task, activity, project and programme of the health management model requires monitoring and mid-term evaluation.

Therefore, evaluation can be understood as continuous and ongoing throughout the management process of the health institution. Follow-up actions should be analysed by senior management, who will develop corrective measures, strategies or reformulate the actions determined to achieve the implementation of the established goals.

An improvement plan will be developed, seeking to implement new activities and strategies to achieve the expected quality assurance from the initial design.

Follow-up and intermediate evaluations must be carried out in each of the phases, tasks, activities, projects and programmes of the Health Management Model.

Evaluation can therefore be understood as continuous and ongoing throughout the entire management process in the health institution.

Continuous improvement plans will be established, which will seek to implement new actions and strategies for further improvement and quality assurance.

FEEDBACK

Any strategy designed in the monitoring process should be disseminated throughout the organisation, restarting in a cyclical and systematic way the whole process of continuous improvement.

Feedback is an imperative when developing a health management system; by sharing specific information about their own performance, the work team will be able to develop the necessary actions to restart a process with new objectives to be developed. It is a constructive and formative process that does not intend to judge or hold the person who performs the procedure or operation responsible, but to learn to build on what has been learned; sharing knowledge. It points out their strengths and weaknesses so that they can use them to plan future practice. Unfortunately, it is an activity that we often skip or fail to do effectively. The lack of culture in the medical community regarding feedback as a key tool to improve the quality of education and health is a pillar of the PLECOSER model.

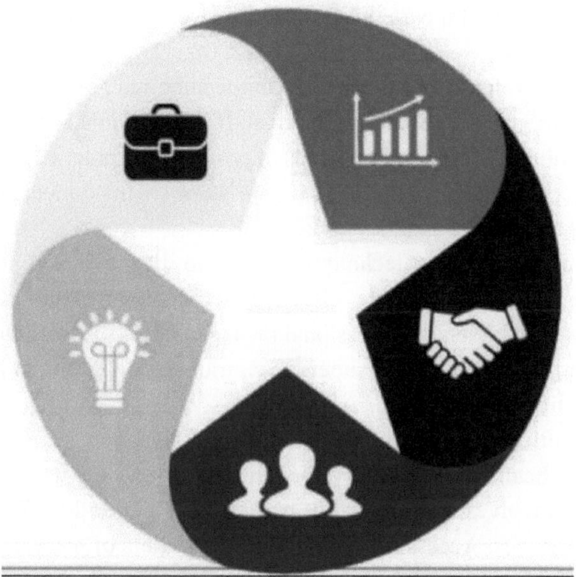

Figure 6. PLECOSER model

DIMENSIONS OF QUALITY

In order to develop the PLECOSER System, it is necessary to be clear about the eight dimensions required for the progress of the system:

Human talent

Accessibility

Effectiveness

Customer Satisfaction

Efficiency

Continuity

Security

Commodities

1. Human talent

Well-educated human capital, regardless of the field or intellectual discipline to which their work activities relate, contributes to the intellectual stock of a country or region and has a significant impact on productivity and development capacity, as a skilled population is an important asset. Change, a creative source of its own resources, creates new knowledge and solves specific problems. It is this reality facing health workers today that is addressed in the World Health Organization's (WHO) World Health Report 2006, which includes an in-depth reflection on the value of human capital in service industries such as health care, where health workers embody the strengths of health care.

Appropriateness refers to the functional competence and performance of health care team, administrative and support staff. Professional preparedness is concerned with implementing standards of professional practice and achieving reliability, accuracy, dependability and consistency. This dimension relates to both clinical and non-clinical services.

In healthcare, this includes techniques related to diagnosis and treatment, as well as the ability to provide effective health counselling and develop relationships with patients. Professional management skills require the highest level of compliance in terms of supervision, training and problem solving.

2. Accessibility

Access to health actions and services represents the patient's ability to obtain, when needed, health care in a convenient manner.

Accessibility involves the removal of barriers that hinder the effective use of health care services. Accessibility is limited by barriers of nature:

• Geographic. Geographic access includes distances, means of transport, travel time and any other physical barriers that prevent the client from receiving care.

• Economic. Refers to the economic ease of obtaining the products and services offered to customers.

• Social or cultural. This relates to the acceptability of the services offered, taking into account cultural values and social attitudes.

• Organisational. This refers to the extent to which the organisation of services is convenient for potential clients; clinic hours and shift systems, waiting time and mode of service delivery are examples of how the organisation of services can create barriers to service use. For example, the lack of evening clinics may present an organisational barrier for day workers. In a society where people cannot easily travel to the health centre, the lack of services in the community or routine home visits can create a problem of access.

• Linguistic. Linguistic access means that services are presented in a language that allows clients to easily express themselves and understand the health worker.

3. Effectiveness

The quality of health services depends on the effectiveness of service delivery standards and clinical guidelines. Effectiveness assessment should answer the questions: When is the treatment delivered correctly, does it produce the desired results, and is the recommended treatment and the technology used the most appropriate for the setting in which the service is provided?

Human resources play an important role in the effectiveness of administrative and service systems in health, especially in terms of their values and motivation.

The mission in health institutions is to provide adequate care to patients in a timely and efficient manner, specialised in the care area and in the administrative processes as well.

It is unquestionable that human talent is the fundamental pillar of the public health system in any country, with an impact on the quality and access to services by the population, thus guaranteeing the coverage of their rights.

Effectiveness in the management of health organisations is understood as the degree to which objectives are met, and is strongly related to the quality perceived by users, and is an important dimension of quality at the central level where standards and specifications are defined. Effectiveness issues are also important to consider at the local level as managers decide how to implement standards and adapt them to local conditions. When determining which standards should be applied in a given situation, the relative risks involved in a population with a high number of high-risk pregnancies, the more frequent use of caesarean section may be justified, despite the associated risks. To determine whether this is an effective strategy, the danger avoided by the procedure must be weighed against the net benefits, taking into account the associated complications.

4. Customer satisfaction

The user satisfaction dimension refers to the relationship between providers and clients, between managers and health service providers, and between the health service team and the community. Good interpersonal relationships contribute to the effectiveness of the health care provided and to the establishment of a good overall relationship with patients. Such relationships are those that build trust and credibility, and are demonstrated through respect, confidentiality, courtesy, understanding and rapport.

The way of listening and communicating is also an important aspect. Health services can be delivered in a professionally competent manner, but if interpersonal relationships are inadequate, there is a risk that care will be less effective. For example, if the patient is not treated well, he or she may not follow the recommendations made by the health team member, or may not get the care needed in the future because he or she feels uncomfortable with the way he or she was treated. Thus, problems in the client satisfaction dimension may compromise the overall quality of care.

Health service user satisfaction surveys are a health care quality indicator that ultimately evaluates the outcome of the health care system, its process and structure; determining the level of satisfaction will make it possible to improve shortcomings and reaffirm strengths in order to develop a health care system that provides the quality care that patients demand.

5. Efficiency

Efficiency of health services is an important dimension of quality given that health care resources are generally limited. Efficient services are those that provide *optimal* patient and community care; that is, they provide the greatest benefit within the resources available. Efficiency requires that health care providers avoid providing unnecessary or inappropriate care and that substandard care that results from ineffective standards is minimised or eliminated. In addition to causing unnecessary risk and patient discomfort, substandard care is often expensive and time-consuming to correct. Two ways to improve quality would be to eliminate waste and avoid errors while reducing costs . However, it would be misleading to imply that quality improvements never require additional resources. Some improvements cost money. Through an efficiency analysis, health programme managers can determine the most cost-effective way to use additional resources.

We health professionals are specialists in converting subjective concepts into measurable parameters, we order and classify them. A health system is considered efficient when it is able to provide a health product acceptable to society with a minimum use of resources. Achieving efficiency in health also means achieving the best results with the available resources.

6. Continuity

Continuity implies that the user of the system receives a full range of health services that he or she requires without unnecessary interruptions, suspensions or repetitions of assessment, diagnosis or treatment. Services should be offered on an ongoing basis. In addition, the client should have access to routine and preventive care from a provider who knows his or her medical history, so that timely referrals to specialised services can be made when appropriate. Sometimes, continuity is achieved by ensuring that clients visit the same primary care provider; in other situations, it is achieved by maintaining well-ordered and archived medical records, so that a new member of the health care team knows the patient's medical history and can build on and complement the diagnosis and treatment of previous providers. Continuity is a very important dimension of quality health care services and its lack can compromise effectiveness, reduce the quality of client satisfaction and decrease the efficiency of care.

Ideally, there should be continuity of health professionals, so that medical care is provided to the individual in a coordinated and uninterrupted manner, despite the complexity of the health system and the involvement of different professionals from different health fields.

7. Security

Safety, as a dimension of quality, implies the reduction of risks, infections, harmful side effects or other hazards that may be associated with the provision of services. It is the conscious attempt to avoid injury to the patient caused by care, is an essential component of Quality of Care and the precondition for the performance of any clinical activity. Safety is a concern of all members of the health care team as well as the patient. The health system has a responsibility to ensure that services are provided with a minimum of risk. Patients must be protected from infection and health workers who handle blood and syringes must also be protected by setting and using safe procedures.

While safety seems to be of greater importance in the provision of complex clinical services, there are also safety issues in the provision of basic health services. For example, waiting rooms in health facilities can expose patients to infection if measures are not taken to prevent it. If a health worker does not provide proper instructions for the preparation of an oral rehydration solution (ORS), a mother may administer an ORS containing a dangerously high concentration of salt to her child.

The safety culture in health care institutions establishes the set of values and norms common to individuals within the same organisation and implies a shared model that positions safety as a priority and common objective to be pursued.

8. Commodities

Hotel amenities refer to those features of health services that are not directly related to clinical effectiveness, but which increase client satisfaction and their desire to return to the facility for future care. Amenities are also important because they can influence patient expectations and confidence in other aspects of the service or product.

In addition, when considering cost recovery, amenities may serve to make patients more willing to pay for services. Amenities often relate to the physical appearance of the facility, staff and materials; as well as physical comforts, cleanliness and privacy. For example, a waiting room that is comfortable, has comfortable seating and pleasant décor, clean and easily accessible restrooms, and consultation rooms that provide privacy. All of these represent some amenities that may be important to patients.

Other amenities may include features that make waiting more pleasant, such as music, educational videos and reading materials. While some amenities are considered luxuries in health facilities in many developing countries, they are nevertheless important for attracting and maintaining client relationships, as well as for ensuring continuity and coverage of services.

Diagnosis of the Quality Assurance System

Questions	**Yes**	**No**	**Not applicable**
1. Have you gone through the qualification process?			
2. Has the hospital management established its strategic vision and do all levels of the company understand the mission?			
3. Is management successfully using the quality management system to achieve its strategic objectives?			
Is management effectively using a quality system that meets the requirements of its customers, its patients, its employees?			
5. Does the quality system in place allow you to "say what you do, do what you say and act to correct differences"?			
6. Do we know who our customers are?			
7. Do we understand what our customers want?			
8. Do we agree with our customers on what is needed?			
9. Do we have the capacity to deliver the services our client needs?			
10. Do we have an adequate way of planning how to design operations and the steps we need to take to execute and control our service processes?			
11. Do we have procedures, manuals, guides, work instructions, etc. to help us carry out our work?			
12. Are we confident that our procedures accurately describe how we do our work?			
13. Are the procedures and work instructions available, are they useful to those who need them, and are these items used?			
Questions	**Yes**	**No**	**Not**

			applicable
14. Do we know if all employees have the latest updated version of the required procedures and work instructions?			
15. Is the documentation we use reviewed and authorised for application by knowledgeable and responsible persons?			
16. Do our suppliers understand and know our needs?			
17. Are our suppliers able to provide the products and services we need?			
18. Are we taking care of things like our patient, products, services, or information that our customer gives us and that we use in the service we provide?			
19. Do we identify, document, assess and inform the affected patient when we have a failure?			
20. When something is identified as an error, does the responsible person ensure that the problem has been resolved?			
21. Do we know and handle complaints and comments from our users in an effective and efficient way?			
22. Can we carefully handle, store, package, persevere and deliver the physical components of our service (laboratory samples, documents, results) in such a way that they reach our customer undamaged?			
23. Can we protect our staff as they handle, package, store, preserve and deliver the physical components of our service?			
24. Do we have indicators that can demonstrate that we have been successful in our work?			
25. Are basic records (medical history, certificates) digitised, legible and usable?			
Questions	**Yes**	**No**	**Not applicable**
26. Do we have the back-up of our records and can we easily consult them when we need them?			
27. Are we effectively using a continuous feedback process to maintain and improve our work processes?			
28. Are we able to demonstrate with certainty that "we say what we do and do what we say"?			
29. Is there a process in place to conduct systems and			

compliance evaluations and demonstrate that a quality assurance programme is helping our health institution to achieve its strategic objectives?			
30. Do we know what professional training and experience our staff need to perform their work successfully?			
31. Do we provide adequate ongoing training to ensure that our staff have the necessary expertise to carry out their activities?			
32. If we need it, can we identify our service quickly, its components and how it should be used?			
33. Can we reconstruct the delivery of a service?			
34. Is the procedure for handling medical records documented and complied with?			
35. Do we know what we are doing and how the work is done?			
36. Are we consistently delivering excellent customer service through our ability to control the internal process?			
37. Is the institutional medical audit carried out?			
Questions	**Yes**	**No**	**Not applicable**
38. Do we know what we need to do to receive products and services at our health facility and are we doing it?			
39. Do all our employees review their work as they perform it and before passing it on to the next person in the service chain?			
40. Before we finish the service, do we confirm if it is well done?			
41. Do we know what we need to measure and do we have the measurement equipment we need to deliver our services adequately?			
42. Do we know if our equipment is capable of measuring what we need it to measure?			
43. Do we know whether our measuring equipment is working accurately as we expect it to, i.e. is it calibrated properly?			
44. Have we carefully reviewed the steps necessary to deliver the services, identifying checkpoints to ensure that the work is being done satisfactorily?			

45. Do we know if a step in our service process has been completed or performed correctly before starting the next step in the process?			
46. If something is wrong, do we take the necessary actions to ensure that the error does not continue in the process of the work so that it does not come to the detriment of our client?			
47. Do we know the terms of the processes we provide?			
48. Have we identified, do we know and do we effectively use a system of information, measurement, techniques and other statistical tools to evaluate			
Questions	**Yes**	**No**	**Not applicable**
When are we meeting the planned and identified strategic objectives?			
49. If you encounter negative test results, what strategies would you use to achieve compliance with these requirements?			

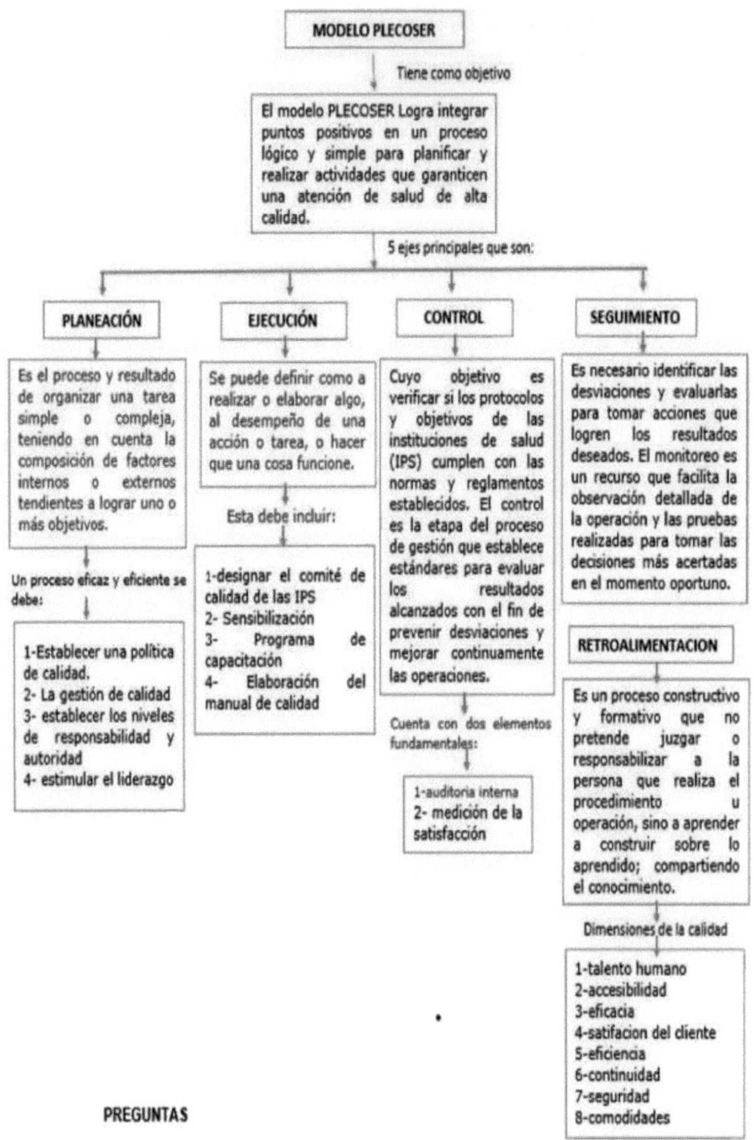

Figure 7. Model for the Development of Health Management Systems

QUESTIONS

1- What is the objective of the Plecoser model?

2- What are the 5 axes that underpin this model?

3- What institutional policies underpin the planning axis?

4- What are the key points to consider for an effective and efficient planning process?

5- How many dimensions should be taken into account in developing the Plecoser system? What are they?

Chapter 6

The User, Epicentre of the Health Management System

"The only way to do a job well is to love what you do. If you haven't found it yet, keep looking. Don't despair. As in love, you'll know when you've found it", Steve Jobs (Speech at Stanford University).

The integrated health management system is based on quality. The word quality originally comes from Latin and its meaning is a characteristic that distinguishes people, goods and services. Although the concept has changed over the years, it has become an important part of the health planning process and clearly implies an effective response to situations affecting the population, the implementation of necessary standards, measures and alternatives, and the use of validation of instruments and medical devices to protect health.

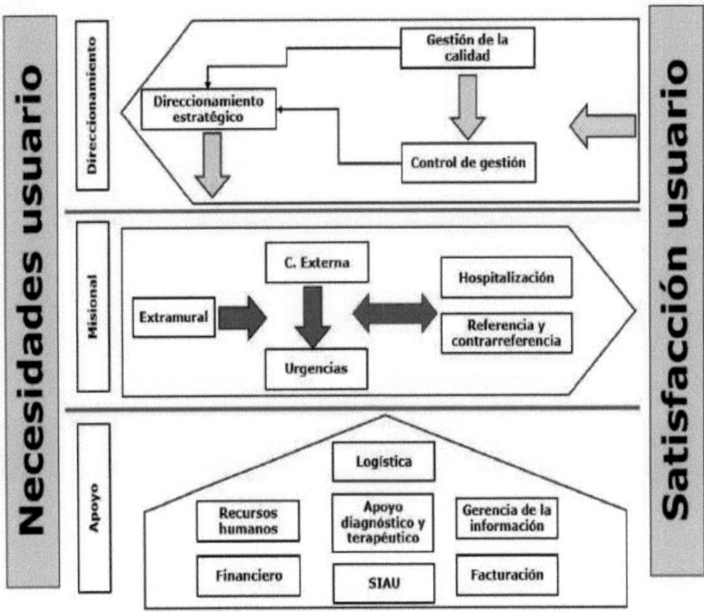

Figure 8. Quality management system

The concept of quality to this day has always represented a challenge, the difference in theoretical conceptions leads to a rainbow of interpretation options and applications, if it is accepted that health care is given in a context of interrelation of processes that makes the products have different levels, which is more complex, so getting to be clear about how to achieve it is an exercise full of experiences and learning that has allowed the development of the PLECOSER model as an applicable methodology to achieve it.

Under this topic in consideration it is important to think that the biological condition of the person is different for each one within their own individuality, therefore, it is that the requirement of the need for care will be transferred within a context of conceptions of care that imposes the health service provider to consider extensively how to achieve that each and every one of them obtains that satisfaction. Many investigations in different countries of the Western world have shown that the degree of quality of care obtained by a user is far from the desired one, and that this difference in the quality of care provided by different health professionals and hospitals is insurmountable, as a condition of multiple factors and situations that occur in health systems.

Thus, the Pan American Health Organisation (PAHO) insinuates that the advancement of Quality Assurance Programmes is necessary in methods of efficiency and an imperative in ethical and moral issues.

It is not possible to talk about quality in health without first being familiar with the ideas conceived by the great visionaries in the field.

For this purpose, the postulates of Steve Jobs, Joseph M. Juran, Walter Shewhart, W. Edwards Deming, Kaoru Ishikawa, Avedis Donabedian, which are considered fundamental in the science of management and the main input for the development of the PLECOSER MODEL, will be reviewed.

Steve Jobs

In Steve Jobs' speech at Stanford University in June 2005, he recalled that when he dropped out of college, he decided to take a calligraphy course at Reed College, which he said then offered "the best calligraphy instruction in the country", because he no longer had to attend the required classes. While it was of no practical use to him at the time, not useful for making money, it was something he was passionate about? He did it and enjoyed it.

Ten years later, when he was designing the first Macintosh computer, Jobs said that "it all made sense" to him: "We designed everything on the Mac. It was the first computer with beautiful typography. Following his instincts gave him an insight that he then applied and became one of his differentiating values.

It is said that before the first launch of the iPod, employees would spend all night changing headphones because Jobs felt they didn't "click" properly and the way he wanted them to. Maintaining quality criteria is fundamental for an entrepreneur, we must not lose sight of what is simple, what is practical or "what sells".

For Jobs, commitment to quality work is fundamental to the development of an idea. You can't leave things half done, settle for "what's there". Aim for more, but don't hold back. It's not about having to produce a perfect product the first time, it's about knowing that everything can be improved. Achieving this is an extremely important differential point.

JOSEPH M. JURAN

Better known as the father of quality, he was born on 24 December 1904 in the city of Braila, Romania. Juran argues that the concept of quality should be taken as the lack of errors or faults that can manifest themselves as: delayed deliveries, faults or errors during the provision of services, erroneous invoices, etc. Therefore, quality is about meeting the needs of the user.

The Juran Trilogy

1. Quality planning. Through planning, it is possible to determine the operational strength in order to realise products that will satisfy the needs of customers or users.
2. Quality control. Processes that are not under strict control are the ones that can show variations, and their impacts can be so enormous that they do not allow analysis of the parts of the process that need to be changed. In order to improve a process, it must first be standardised and under control.
3. Quality improvement. This premise is aimed at modifying the process in order to achieve better levels of quality, and for this it is essential to identify the most significant usual reasons that affect the process.

WALTER SHEWHART

This theorist made two very important points:

- The PH VA cycle. The Plan, Do, Check, Act cycle is a key methodology for continuous improvement processes.
- Statistical process control. It is of great advantage in the monitoring and improvement of processes.

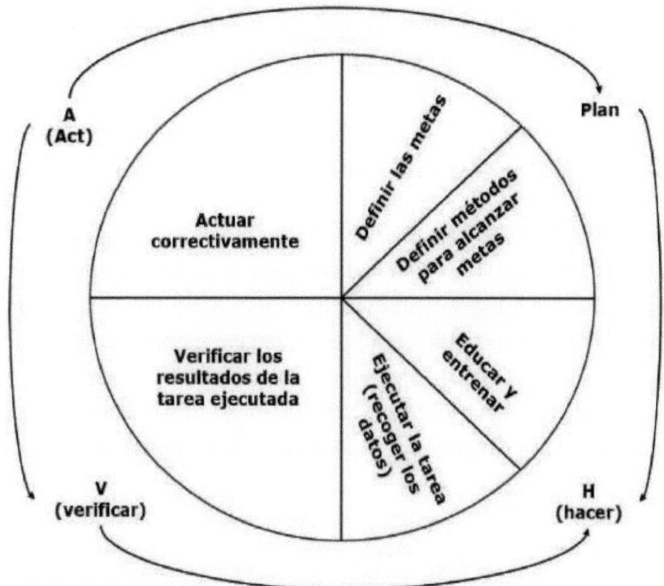

Figure 9. PHVA Cycle

Planning (P). This first phase is composed of two stages. First: Identify goals (what). Second: Define ways to achieve the goals (how).

Doing (H). This is the phase of action or execution of what has already been stipulated in the first phase; it consists of two stages: the first is the training of people; the second is the implementation of what has been planned.

Verify (V). This is the phase of checking or verifying the results.

Act (A). In this fourth or last phase it is necessary to proceed in relation to the whole process. If the goal has been achieved, it is essential to standardise the execution in order to ensure the results of the process. If the goal has not been achieved, there is an urgent need to correct and fine-tune the process, in order to turn the cycle around again until the goal is achieved. Therefore, Figure 6 shows circular arrows, implying that it is a never-ending cycle. It will always be adjusted in the direction of achieving the results.

W. EDWARDS DEMING

Best considered the Father of Modern Quality, he was born on October 14, 1900, in Sioux City, Iowa. His childhood was associated with poverty and hard work. He studied engineering at the University of Wyoming. He received a PhD in Mathematical Physics from Yale University in 1927. He met Walter Shewhart, a statistician who worked for Bell Laboratories, and his writings became the basis of his teachings.

During World War II, he trained American technicians and engineers in statistics so that they could improve the quality of war supplies. It was this work that caught the attention of the Japanese. After the war, the Japanese Union of Scientists and Engineers approached

Deming. He went to Japan in 1950 at the age of 49 and for the next 30 years taught Japanese managers, engineers and scientists how to produce with quality.

It is worth noting that Deming was invited to Japan precisely when its industry and economy were in crisis. They listened carefully and changed their way of thinking, their management style and their treatment of employees. With the concepts proposed in Deming's philosophy, the Japanese completely changed their economy and productivity to become the world market leaders.

It was not until a documentary aired on NBC in June 1980, detailing Japan's industrial success, that American corporations took notice and sought Deming's advice.

Deming shared with some of America's largest corporations his now famous *Fourteen Points* and *Seven Deadly Sins*.

He concluded that the quick and easy solutions typical of corporate America did not work. Through a transformative process of moving forward and following the *Fourteen Points* and *Seven Deadly Sins*, American business would be in a position to keep pace with the constantly changing economic environment.

According to Deming's proposal: Quality is not a luxury; Quality is the predictable degree of uniformity and safety, at a low cost and that suits the market.

If Deming's principles are in place and running with your company, and according to Gonzalez (2007), "quality increases, costs go down and savings can be passed on to the consumer, customers get quality products, companies get higher revenues and the economy grows".

Deming penetrated corporate America in consulting matters and private individuals through manuscripts and seminar tours during 13 years of his life. Although he died in 1993, his work still lives on.

The Deming cycle prepared by Shewhart. It is essentially a method used by companies to improve their processes. It is based on the administrative process divided into four stages:

1. Planning. Projecting a product based on market needs, establishing descriptions and the production process.
2. To do. To carry out the project.
3. Controlling. To verify or control the product according to quality indicators

during the stages of the production and marketing process.

4. Analyse and Update. Decipher reports, records to act through variations in product design, production and commercial processes to achieve continuous improvement.

THE FOURTEEN POINTS

1. To be constant in the purpose of improving products and services.
2. Adopt the new philosophy.
3. No more reliance on mass inspection.
4. End the practice of awarding procurement contracts on the basis of price alone.
5. Continuous and permanent improvement of the production and service system.
6. Institute on-the-job training.
7. Institutionalising leadership.
8. Banish fear.
9. Breaking down barriers between staff areas.
10. Eliminate slogans, exhortations and goals for the workforce.
11. Eliminate numerical quotas.
12. Breaking down the barriers that prevent a sense of pride in a job well done.
13. Establish a vigorous education and retraining programme.
14. Take action to achieve transformation.

THE SEVEN DEADLY SINS

1. Lack of perseverance of purpose.
2. Enhance profits for the short term.
3. Assessing performance.
4. Continuous management change.
5. Managing a company based solely on tangible figures.
6. High sanitation costs.
7. Extraordinary guarantee costs promoted by lawyers working on a fee basis when unforeseen events occur.

KAORU ISHIKAWA

Born in Japan in 1915. Graduated from the Department of Engineering, University of Tokyo. He graduated with a PhD in Engineering from that university. He won the Deming Award and was recognised by the American Quality Association.

He is the first author who sought to establish the differences between Japanese and Western management styles. He is one of the forerunners of the concept of total quality in Japan. As such, he had a strong influence on the rest of the world by highlighting the cultural differences between countries as an important factor in achieving quality success. He is a great believer in the importance of philosophy among Eastern peoples. He is also convinced of the obligation to change the way people think about their work. Quality can be indicated as a constant process that usually could go one step further. Today he is known as one of the world's best-known quality gurus.

Ishikawa implemented his quality control in post-war Japan. He defined it as "developing, designing, manufacturing and maintaining a quality product". Perhaps Ishikawa's most significant contribution was his contribution to a Japanese quality strategy.

Furthermore, he believed that company managers should not only focus on making quality products, but that quality should be present throughout the company, even after purchasing. He was also in favour of quality being taken beyond the work area, into the daily life of each person.

He is one of the founders of the Union of Japanese Scientists and Engineers (UJSE), an association that worked to maintain quality in Japan throughout the post-war period.

Ishikawa made many contributions, including the following:

- First author to use the concept of Total Quality Control (TQC).
- I design the cause-effect diagram, or Ishikawa fishbone diagram.
- He explained the importance of using the 7 quality tools.
- He worked in quality circles. Analysed that quality circles were of greater importance for service companies than for manufacturing companies.

Looking deeper into the Cause-Effect Diagram, it can be reduced to the fact that when analysing any problem, and not only health-related problems, they usually have different causes with different degrees of importance. Some reasons may be related to the beginning of the problem and others to the consequences of the problem.

Therefore, the diagram designed by Ishikawa allows the origins of the problem to be studied or analysed to be plotted. It is known as the "Fishbone" due to due to the way in which each of the origins or causes that, in our opinion, give rise to the problem are placed. Its advantage is that it helps to quickly and clearly observe the relationship between each of the causes with the rest of the reasons that determine the origin of the problem. On certain occasions they may be independent causes and on others, there is a close relationship between them.

It is considered that the best way to identify problems is through the participation of the whole work team and motivating the participants to put forward their suggestions. The ideas or concepts expressed by the members will be placed in different parts of the diagram. This is why the Ishikawa diagram can be deduced by observing the results achieved.

KEY ELEMENTS OF ISHIKAWA THINKING

- Quality starts with education and ends with education.
- The first step towards quality is to determine what the customer needs.
- The ideal stage of quality is when inspection is not needed.
- We need to look at the root of the problem, not the clues.
- Quality control is the responsibility of all employees.
- Do not confuse means with goals.
- Put quality first and then long-term profits.
- Trade is the input and output of quality.
- Senior company executives should not begrudge staff when they provide valuable feedback.
- Problems can be solved with simple tools for analysis. - Information without dissemination information is misinformation.

Kaoru Ishikawa also introduces the world to the seven basic tools such as:

1. Pareto chart.
2. Cause-Effect Diagram.
3. Stratification.
4. Check Sheet.
5. Histogram.
6. Dispersion Diagram.
7. Schewhart Control Chart.

AVEDIS DONABEDIAN

Forerunner of the study of quality in health care and essentially known for his various concepts or pillars of quality. Born in Beirut, Lebanon, on 7 June 1919, he lived in an Arab village north of Jerusalem. He studied medicine at the American University of Beirut and in 1953 he moved to the United States to study for a Masters in Public Health at Harvard University in 1955. In 1961 he became Professor at the School of Public Health at the University of Beirut. Michigan, where he developed the central part of his theories. He died on 9 November 2000.

At the time of his death he was a Professor at Nathan Sinai as Distinguished Professor Emeritus of Public Health. He was also a member of the Institute of Medicine of the National Academy of Sciences of the United States of America and an Honorary Fellow of the Royal College of General Practitioners of the United Kingdom and of the National Academy of Medicine of Mexico. He was awarded the Sedgwick Medal for Distinguished Service in Public Health in 1999, the highest award conferred by the American Public Health Association. Donabedian focused greater attention on the specific issue of quality of care in health care that transformed the models that were in place at the time. Through eight books and more than 50 articles and numerous papers, he changed thinking about health systems. He saw the social response to health difficulties not as a group of unrelated events, but rather as a complicated cause guided by general principles. In the vast majority of his texts Donabedian was ahead of his colleagues, manifesting a broad intellectual horizon.

He is the author who introduced the concepts of Structure, Process and Outcome, which form the prevailing model of health care quality assessment. In the June 2000 issue of the World Health Organisation's bulletin, Donabedian presented one of his texts, in which he discussed the measurement of physician competence. In the introductory part of this article he paid special attention to the effects of quality of care.

There is no denying that Donabedian was a tireless campaigner to try to bridge the gap between academia - theory - and action - practice.

His condition of having prostate cancer since 1972 led him to understand his peers so well, having been a patient himself for many years of his life. The statements he communicated to Fizthugh Mullan a month before he died give us much insight into his thinking about health care.

- "The quality you see in the hospital is really limited to the technical competence and, more recently, to the superficial attention to the interpersonal process. Keep the patient happy, be nice to the patient, call them sir or madam; remember their name. The idea that patients should be involved in their care is generally not practised responsibly. Today people talk about patient autonomy, but that usually translates into patient neglect. The physician must work diligently with the patient in order to arrive at a solution that is ultimately acceptable to the patient, but is not patient-directed. The physician's role is to actively ensure that the patient arrives at a reasonable decision, but without being manipulative.
- "Many doctors hide behind the claim that they are good clinicians but that the system is wrong, not realising that they are the key aspect of the system (...)".
- "There is no system management taught in medical schools or health fields. And then doctors and nurses are put in charge of systems that are often under short-term financial pressures. These pressures are real, but the goal of good systems must be to deal with them.
- "I have never been convinced that competition alone can improve the efficiency or effectiveness of care or even reduce the cost of care. I think the commercialisation of care is a big mistake. Health is a sacred mission. It is a moral enterprise and a scientific enterprise but not a commercial enterprise in

the strict sense. We are not selling a product. We do not have a customer who understands everything and makes reasonable choices - and I include myself in that as well. Doctors and nurses are guides to something very valuable. Their work is a kind of vocation and not just a job; commercial values do not capture what they do for patients and for society as a whole.

• "Systems awareness and systems design are important for health professionals, but they are not enough. They are only enabling mechanisms. What is essential for the success of a system is the ethical dimension of individuals. Ultimately, the secret of quality is love. One must love one's patient; one must love one's profession; one must love one's God. If you have love, then you can look back to monitor and improve the system. Commercialism should not be the central force in the system".

Other important but less known thinkers include: Philip B. Crosby, Genichi Taguchi, Shigeo Shingo, Jan Carlzon, Stephen R. Covey, Taiichi Ohno, Masaka Imai, we highlight below their most important contributions.

PHILIP B. CROSBY

Crosby argues that quality is based on four absolute principles:

1. Quality is meeting the requirements
2. The quality system is prevention
3. The standard of performance is zero defects
4. The measure of quality is the price of non-compliance.

Derived from the above principles, his proposal is for a 14-step programme to improve quality:

1. Management commitment
2. Quality improvement team
3. Measuring the level of quality
4. Quality awareness
5. Assessing the cost of quality
6. Corrective action system
7. Establish Zero Defects Programme Committee
8. Supervisory training
9. Set Zero Defect Day
10. Setting goals
11. Remove causes of errors
12. Giving recognition
13. Forming quality councils
14. Repeat all over again

Every company that is based on quality management goes through six phases of change called the 6Cs:

1. Compression
2. Commitment
3. Competition
4. Communication
5. Correction
6. Continuity

But, the administration has the responsibility to deliver the three T's:

1. Weather
2. Talent
3. Treasury

On the other hand, Crosby devised the quality vaccine, which represents the need for every company to report non-conforming product in accordance with product specifications. Therefore, the vaccine is made up of the following elements:

- Integrity
- Systems
- Communications
- Operations
- Policies

GENICHI TAGUSHI

Another author who is a little known is Genichi Tagushi. This author defines quality in terms of economic loss. Therefore, quality is defined in monetary form through the loss function, whereby the greater the variation of a specification in relation to the nominal value, the greater the economic loss passed on to the consumer.

The 7 points of TAGUSHI

1. It is important to define quality in economic terms through the loss function.
2. In order to survive today, it is necessary to apply the process of continuous improvement and the reduction of variability as they are indispensable.
3. The process of continuous improvement is closely related to the reduction of variability focused on the target value.
4. Variability in product performance creates a loss to the user and this can be valued as the square of the difference between the actual performance and the plotted value.
5. It is through the design phase that the quality is established and the final cost of the product is estimated.
6. A product can be designed based on the non-linear part of its response in order to reduce variability.
7. Variability can be reduced through the design of experiments by choosing

the ideal types of variables involved in product manufacture.

Therefore, quality engineering performs tasks with the aim of reducing the losses caused by variation.

SHIGEO SHINGO

He is an author who is possibly better known for his contributions in the area of production maximisation than total quality. However, the main thesis for his philosophy is that one of the biggest obstacles to maximising production is encountering quality difficulties. His SMED method works wonders if you have a zero-defect process, for which he proposed the development of Poka-Yoke (error-proof) systems.

ZERO INVENTORIES

One of the advantages that a company can gain from the zero in-process inventory method, in addition to the financial savings, are:

Drastic reduction of production defects to zero, due to the fact that when a defect occurs, production is stopped until the causes of the defect can be eliminated. Therefore, by reducing defects to zero, the surplus of raw materials due to rejected products is reduced to zero and the consumption of energy and other consumable materials is reduced to a minimum.

In addition, factories require less space because they do not have to store in-process inventories or irregular or defective materials.

Thus, the production system is obliged to work flawlessly, which makes it predictable and therefore safe in relation to just-in-time delivery.

Therefore, the POKA-YOKE system is nothing more than the development of units that help to detect production defects and report them promptly in order to get to the root of the problem and prevent it from happening again.

Shingo also proposed the concept of source review to find errors in time. Through this method, the process is stopped and corrected immediately in order to prevent it from turning into a defective product at a later stage.

Another factor for success in the production process is the implementation of the Five S's: which stands for order and cleanliness. This is made possible by organising the workplace by introducing the Japanese 5 S's technique:

1. Seri: Selection. Differentiating what is necessary from what is not.
2. Seition: Order. A place for everything and everything in its place.
3. Seiso: Cleanliness. Use methods to keep the workplace clean.
4. Seiketsu: Standardisation. Establish standards and methods that are easy to follow.
5. Shitsuke: Maintenance. Create methods to make it a habit.

POKA-YOKE PREVENTION LEVELS

The levels of prevention indicated for Poka-Yoke include:

Level Zero. Provide minimum information to employees about normal operations.
Level 1. Reporting the results of control activities. Report the results of control activities so that each employee can observe his or her performance.
Level 2. Standards information. Standards and methods are indicated so that each employee can begin to find non-conformities and help to correct them.
Level 3. Establish clear standards within the workplace. Make a standard of your own working environment, with its materials, equipment or space, build normal methods and processes into your own workplace.
Level 4. Alarms. To guide inspection time and speed of response, it is necessary to install a visible alarm to indicate to employees when a defect or irregularity has occurred.
Level 5. Prevention. The visual monitoring system provides the necessary time and subtlety to detect and correct irregularities.
Level 6. Error-proofing. The use of a wide range of devices to inspect 100 per cent of the products so that they are designed to be error or failure proof, and to ensure that the irregularity will not recur during the process.

JAN CARLZON

This author is credited with the concept of *moments of truth*, from which a whole quality management programme for service companies was developed. For Carlzon, moments of truth are those intervals of time in which a company's employees have contact with its customers to carry out the delivery of a service, it is during these moments that the company is put to the test, as the image depends at these moments on the employee's ability to satisfy the customer's needs and to make a good impression.

Within its quality strategy, all the steps that the customer follows at the moment of receiving the service are detailed, from the customer's point of view, this is called the service cycle and it establishes the moments of truth that can be found, who is in charge at those moments and what must be known or decided in order to accept responsibilities.

He called the process of transferring authority to make decisions about company policies and regulations *empowerment*. According to Carlzon, all employees need to feel and know that they are needed, as motivation is a fundamental key to achieving quality.

Whereas, customers are not interested in knowing that they are part of a large employer-identified market, they all want to be treated as individuals, so the customer service employee should not feel committed to company policies designed to treat all customers equally. Only that employee will be able to see the differences between customers and will be able to make decisions to provide the customer with what he or she requires.

STEPHEN R. COVEY

According to Covey, habits are the result of being able to intercept knowledge, capacity (ability) and desire (attitude), as these are necessary to achieve personal excellence. He also argues that personal maturity is always in development.

Covey recommends encouraging seven habits that effective people have:

1. Be proactive. Our behaviour is a function of our decisions, not our situations.
2. Have a goal in mind. That is to say, to have a fixed objective, to know where we want to get to.
3. Establish first things first. Know how to self-manage, and not let them do things for us.
4. Think win/win. Consider the win/win relationship, or in other words that both parties are satisfied.
5. Seek first to understand and then to be understood. To do this, empathy must be practised.
6. Synergise. To be able to work in a team.
7. Sharpen the axe. Always strive for continuous personal excellence.

Looking at these seven points, the first three lead to individual excellence, the next three to social excellence and the last one is the one that makes the previous six possible.

In order to improve you need to be in self-control, you must:

- Knowing where we are going
- Realise whether we are achieving it
- Having the means and the opportunities to achieve it

As can be deduced from the above, the achievement of quality is an approach that goes hand in hand with the concept of health service delivery. We must be aware, convinced and committed to develop all our actions and strategies within the framework of achieving user satisfaction, efficient service delivery, and thus generating the lowest possible costs.

To do this, we must generate, ensure, control and improve our processes, framed in the full satisfaction of our internal and external users. Develop a management system based on processes.

TAIICHI OHNO

Another of the authors who issued a concept related to quality is Taiichi Ohno. As vice-president of Toyota Motor, he was the creator of the *Just in Time* (JIT) management method. This management method is oriented towards improving the company's results with the participation of all employees by eliminating activities that do not add value to the process.

MASAKA IMAI

This Japanese author proposes the Kaizen strategy. It is a system that summarises several theories that can be applied to different company structures. Kaisen is a Japanese word meaning improvement. Its root, Kai, is change and Zen, is goodness. Therefore, for this author, everything can be improved, with the help and participation of all the people involved in the process.

The thoughts of these important thinkers and generators of quality, especially the postulates of Avedis Donabedian, are basic to quality management in health and serve as a foundation for the audit and quality management model presented in the chapter of the PLECOSER Model.

General Health Administration Students' Contribution to this Chapter

It provides an in-depth and comprehensive overview of the concept of quality in health management and its relationship to user satisfaction. Throughout the chapter, the importance of quality is highlighted and different visions and theories of key figures in quality management are presented, including Steve Jobs, Joseph M. Juran, Walter Shewhart, W. Edwards Deming, Kaoru Ishikawa, and Avedis Donabedian.

The chapter begins with a quote from Steve Jobs that emphasises the need to love what you do in order to do it well. This idea of passion and commitment is essential in quality management in healthcare, as healthcare professionals must be fully committed to continuously improving their services to meet the needs of users.

Here, constructive criticism is made of the chapter. While the focus on quality is essential, it would be beneficial to explore further how healthcare institutions can cultivate this passion and commitment among their staff. What support structures, incentives and professional development opportunities can they put in place to motivate their staff to pursue excellence in patient care?

The chapter also approaches the concept of quality from a variety of theoretical perspectives, which adds valuable depth and complexity to the discussion. However, it would be useful to have more synthesis and critical evaluation of these theories: how do these theories compare and contrast, and what practical implications do they have for quality management in health?

Furthermore, while the chapter touches on the importance of individuality and differences in health care needs, it does not explore in depth how health systems can adapt to these differences. How can health systems be designed to be more user-centred and responsive to the individual needs of each patient?

The chapter also emphasises the importance of individuality in healthcare and how health systems need to adapt to the individual needs of each patient. This is a critical aspect of the health management system that is often overlooked, and the discussion on this topic in this chapter is a valuable reminder that each patient is unique and that health systems need to be flexible and adaptable to meet their individual needs.

Furthermore, I find the proposal to use the PLECOSER model as a methodology to achieve quality in healthcare interesting. However, the explanation and description of this model in the chapter could have been more in-depth and detailed so that readers can fully understand how this model can be applied in practice.

In summary, this chapter provides a comprehensive and well-grounded overview of quality management in healthcare, with a strong emphasis on the importance of user-centredness. However, it could benefit from further exploration of how these theoretical concepts of quality can be applied in practice in the health system and how the user experience can be improved.

The chapter provides a broad overview of quality in health management and its impact on user satisfaction. Particularly relevant is the inclusion of different theories and views of key quality management stakeholders. However, it would be useful to provide a more detailed discussion on how these theories can be effectively applied in a healthcare setting.

Although the chapter does a good job of highlighting the importance of passion and commitment in health management, it would benefit from including suggestions or strategies

Can specific incentives or professional development programmes be introduced to promote continuous improvement?

Furthermore, although the chapter mentions the importance of individuality and differences in health care needs, it would be valuable to explore further how health systems can adapt to these differences. How can health systems be designed to be more user-centred and personalise care according to the individual needs of each patient?

The PLECOSER model is presented as an interesting proposal for achieving quality in healthcare. However, it would benefit from a more detailed description and a clearer explanation of how this model can be applied in practice.

In summary, Chapter 6 provides a valuable overview of quality management in health, highlighting the importance of user-centredness. However, it could benefit from more practical details and real-world examples of how these concepts can be implemented in the health system. It would also be useful to include more strategies and suggestions on how to promote passion and

commitment among health staff and how to adapt health systems to meet the individual needs of each patient.
provides an in-depth and comprehensive overview of the concept of quality in healthcare management and its relationship to user satisfaction. Throughout the chapter, the importance of quality is highlighted and different visions and theories of key figures in quality management are presented, including Steve Jobs, Joseph M. Juran, Walter Shewhart, Edwards Deming, Kaoru Ishikawa, and Avedis Donabedian.
The chapter begins with a quote from Steve Jobs that emphasises the need to love what you do in order to do it well. This idea of passion and commitment is essential in quality management in healthcare, as healthcare professionals must be fully committed to continuously improving their services to meet the needs of users.
Here, constructive criticism is made of the chapter. While the focus on quality is essential, it would be beneficial to explore further how healthcare institutions can cultivate this passion and commitment among their staff. What support structures, incentives and professional development opportunities can they put in place to motivate their staff to pursue excellence in patient care?
The chapter also approaches the concept of quality from a variety of theoretical perspectives, which adds valuable depth and complexity to the discussion. However, it would be useful to have more synthesis and critical evaluation of these theories: how do these theories compare and contrast, and what practical implications do they have for quality management in health?
Furthermore, while the chapter touches on the importance of individuality and differences in health care needs, it does not explore in depth how health systems can adapt to these differences. How can health systems be designed to be more user-centred and responsive to the individual needs of each patient?
The chapter also emphasises the importance of individuality in healthcare and how health systems need to adapt to the individual needs of each patient. This is a critical aspect of the health management system that is often overlooked, and the discussion on this topic in this chapter is a valuable reminder that each patient is unique and that health systems need to be flexible and adaptable to meet their individual needs.
Furthermore, I find the proposal to use the PLECOSER model as a methodology to achieve quality in healthcare interesting. However, the explanation and description of this model in the chapter could have been more in-depth and detailed so that readers can fully understand how this model can be applied in practice.
In summary, this chapter provides a comprehensive and well-grounded

overview of quality management in healthcare, with a strong emphasis on the importance of user-centredness. However, it could benefit from further exploration of how these theoretical concepts of quality can be applied in practice in the health system and how the user experience can be improved.

Chapter 7

Observation and Quality

"Tell me how you measure and I'll tell you how I behave".
ELIYAHU M. GOLDRATT

The Hawthorne effect is a result described by psychological science that refers to how the observation of a person during the working day affects their performance. The concept stems from experiments conducted at the Hawthorne Works company, which requested a series of studies within its facilities in order to find out how different types of observation could affect the productivity of each of its employees.

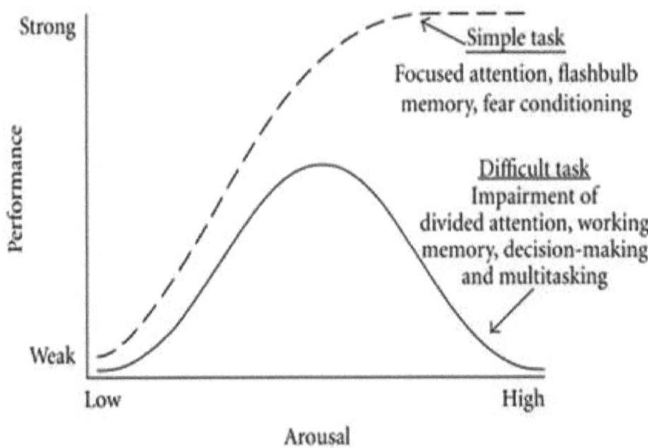

Figure *10.* Results of experiments at Hawthorne Company

The data obtained did not produce much interest until, in the 1950s, researcher Henry Landsberger found that workers' compliance was related to observation. They improved when they felt observed.
According to Landsberger's findings, a large part of the company's staff altered their routines and the intensity of their activity when under direct observation and with prior notice.
The health care model must take into account the Hawthorne effect in the most positive and motivating way, including it in the daily processes for all health care institutions; understanding the desired quality as a set of guidelines, processes, actions and tools applied in the organisation of service provision to guarantee the availability, accessibility, timeliness, acceptability, acceptability, comprehensiveness, quality and professional competence, continuity, strong resolution and efficiency of health care, with a focus on the person and health outcomes, considering their life course and their

environment, in the promotion, prevention, diagnosis, treatment, rehabilitation and palliation that legitimise the fundamental right to health.

The concept of quality has evolved over time, in the past it was tied to the realisation of doing things well regardless of cost or effort, with the aim of producing a unique product. It was more of a craftsmanship type of concept.

With the advent of the industrial revolution, production is linked to quality, the aim is to satisfy demand and thus achieve an economic return.

During the Second World War, quality was related to the effectiveness of armaments without regard for their cost, with the largest and most accelerated production.

In the post-war period, quality in Japan is related to producing things well, minimising costs through quality, satisfying customer requirements. While in the rest of the countries they were characterised by producing more, satisfying the post-war demand.

After this stage, production review techniques began to be introduced to prevent the release of defective products. From this moment on, the concept of quality control was born.

The concept of Quality Assurance is introduced later and is defined as systems developed to prevent imperfect products from being manufactured. Later the concept evolves into what is called Total Quality, a management theory focused on the continuous satisfaction of customer requirements.

Quality of Health Care

Dr. Donabedian has defined quality in health as: "A property of medical care that can be obtained in varying degrees. Obtaining greater benefits with less risk to the user, depending on available resources and prevailing social values. In addition:

Medical care is given as the treatment provided by a health professional to a clearly established episode of illness in a given patient, from which two aspects originate, the first as technical care, which is the application of science and technology for the resolution of a health problem, and the second as the interpersonal relationship, which is the social and economic interaction between the health professional and the patient. (p. 6).

Quality, on the other hand, comprises four dimensions:

1. The technical dimension. It lies in the best implementation of all professional knowledge combined with technology in accordance with procedures and equipment that can be used for the benefit of the patient.
2. Safety. It seeks to ensure that in treating a patient, the greatest benefit is achieved with the least risk to the patient, so that benefits to a patient cannot be achieved at the cost of increased risk to the patient or their relatives.

3. Service. The timeliness and continuity with which patient care is provided is considered to be of utmost importance, with the interpersonal relationship with the patient, the conditions of the place where the service is provided and the easy access available for the provision of the service being very relevant.
4. Cost-benefit ratio. Understanding the relationship between the benefits and risks involved, since improving quality may increase costs.

The concept of quality may vary, depending on the approach from which it is viewed, the interest of the service provider (IPS, professional), the payer (EPS, ARS, patient) or the receiver (user). Juran defines it as "suitability or fitness for use", while for Ishikawa it is "satisfaction of the requirements of the consumers of that product or service".

In institutions where health services are provided, it is necessary to develop quality assurance programmes, starting from the individual clinical service all the way up to the networks of health service providers. It is therefore indispensable to develop continuous procedures for quantitative and qualitative measurement and evaluation of the quality of care provided. To this end, it is essential to establish standards that allow a constant comparison between the system and the perception of the users, with the aim of implementing continuous improvement processes that help to improve quality within the system and for the users of the system.

One of the methods to be able to evaluate the quality of care is through the definition of indicators and standards, as these must be adapted and established according to the particular situation to be evaluated and the objectives sought, because the great challenge for health systems to develop an appropriate evaluation methodology adapted to the needs and opportunities of different areas lies in defining unified criteria about what health care consists of.

Following Dr. Donabedian's teachings, three main elements are taken into account in order to assess quality in health.

1. Structure. These are the characteristics of the areas where care is provided. The purpose of its evaluation is to analyse the particularities of the facilities, equipment, technology, technical and auxiliary human talent, financial resources and internal and external information system. The structure is very important for the development of the processes and for the standards of behaviour of the people and systems included in it. The advantages of this assessment are based on the possibility of being able to obtain objective, valuable and reliable information. Its great disadvantage lies in not being able to deduce the quality of the structure, or the good quality of care. Structure implies the qualities of the facilities in which care takes place. This includes the qualities of the material resources (such as facilities, equipment and

money), of the human resources (number and qualifications of staff), and of the organisational structure (such as the organisation of the medical team, methods of quality control and methods of reimbursement).

2. The process. This involves all the actions performed by the care providers and their skills to deliver care. Quality assessment at the *Process* level incorporates all the information on the services offered by the institution's professionals, and on the extent of coordination and integration between the different departments responsible for diagnosis, treatment and rehabilitation, and of administrative and financial support, where the existence and application of diagnostic and therapeutic management guidelines or protocols is most important. The process involves what is actually done in giving and receiving care. It includes the activities of the patient in seeking and carrying out care and the activities of the practitioner in making a diagnosis and recommending or implementing treatment.

3. Outcomes. These are considered to be the benefits achieved by the patient. The evaluation of the quality of the *results* is measured by means of indicators that assess the preservation or improvement in the patient's state of health, the presence or absence of adverse events, death or disability at different levels. The satisfaction achieved by the provider and the user of the services is also evaluated. The advantages that can be achieved with this evaluation are the effectiveness of health care, that the results in global terms are more real and the quantification more accurate, and the studies can become more universal and comparable with reference to the validity and reliability of those results. The outcome involves the effects of care on patient and population health status. Improvements in patient knowledge and changes in patient health behaviour are included in a broad definition of health status, as is the degree of patient satisfaction with care. . This tripartite approach to quality assessment is only possible because a good structure increases the likelihood of a good process, and a good process increases the likelihood of a good outcome. Therefore, it is necessary to have such a relationship established before any component of structure, process or outcome can be used to assess quality. The activity of quality assessment is not

specifically designed to establish the presence of these relationships. There must be prior knowledge of the relationship between structure and process, and between process and outcome, before quality assessment can be carried out.

The main tool for assessing the quality of health care is the medical audit, which evaluates the structure, processes and results of health service provision. Donabedian is the most expressive on the methodology, which must be kept in mind in order to assess quality. The structure-directed requirements encapsulate the resources available to health care providers; the process parameters comprise the primary object of assessment, including the activities to be performed by and between professionals and patients; and the outcome requirements include the change in the current and future state of the patient's health.

In Colombia, after the implementation of the SGSSS, great emphasis has been placed on the quality of the health services that must be offered by the Service Providing Institutions (IPS), especially with Decree 2174 of 1996, which ordered the Mandatory System of Quality Assurance, subsequently changed by Decree 2309 of 2002 and Decree 1011 of 2006, dated 3 April 2006. Decree 780 of 2016 "Whereby the Sole Regulatory Decree of the Health and Social Protection Sector is issued", which was a compilation of Decree 1011 of 2006 "Whereby the Obligatory System of Quality Assurance of Health Care (SOGCS) of the General System of Social Security in Health is established".

By means of Resolution 3100 of 2019 "Whereby the procedures and conditions for the registration of health service providers and the authorisation of health services are defined and the Manual for the Registration of Health Service Providers and Authorisation of Health Services is adopted".

The SOGCS is composed of four major elements, namely: Sistema Único de Habilitación (SUH), Programa de Auditoria para el Mejoramiento de la Calidad (PAMEC), Sistema Único de Acreditación (SUA) and the Sistema de Información para la Calidad en Salud (SICS).

Summarising, about the fundamental elements to be kept in mind when the system is to be developed, not only as a presentation model but also as a model for the orientation of the public offer at territorial level that supports the provision of health services in the territory and makes the care of the population possible.

Single Enabling System

- Enabling services
- Functional organisations
- Comprehensive networks of health care providers

Single Accreditation System

- Quality Information System
- Quality Improvement Audit

The Obligatory System of Quality Assurance in Health Care aims to protect the health of the population by making possible the rights to life and health enshrined in our Constitution.

Table 2. Structure of health care in Colombia

Administrative	Political strategies

	Leadership
	Goals, objectives
	Administrative procedures
	Reward and recognition systems
	Management methods
	Products, services and specifications
Technique Structure	Technology Know-how
	Information systems
	Equipment, infrastructure
	Skills, knowledge Values, codes of conduct
Humana	Authority and responsibility Division of tasks and functions Mental models
	Standards and rules

Law 100 of 1993 establishes that one of the principles of the public health service is quality in Article 153, Section 9, and relates it to evaluation and control procedures for health services that ensure quality contexts, in the form of timely, personalised, humanised, comprehensive and continuous care, in accordance with national standards and procedures in professional practice.

In addition to establishing Quality as a principle of the SGSSS, Articles 186, 199, 227 and 232 of Law 100 of 1993 provide for the regulation of the Accreditation System to provide information to users on the quality of health service provision and to promote its improvement, as well as to define standards to evaluate user satisfaction, maximum waiting times for services, according to pathologies and user needs. Articles 227 and 232 establish the obligatory nature of the Quality Assurance and Auditing Systems that the IPS and EPS must follow, in order to guarantee the strict quality in the provision of services.

The National Superintendence of Health issued the following circulars with reference to quality:

- External Circular No.014 of 28 December 1995, on Emergency Care.
- External Circular No.022 of 13 November 1996, on the competencies of the Departmental Level on Inspection, Surveillance and Control (IVC) of the SGSSS, which establishes the activities of inspection, control and surveillance of quality in the provision of health services, seeking to verify that the providers of the Public Health Service carry out their activities according to the legal framework that regulates them, especially in compliance with the guiding principles of the General System of Social Security in Health, contained in Law 100 of 1993, among which is Quality.

With the issuance of Law 715 of 21 December 2001, the mandate of Law 100 of 1993 was confirmed and the adjustment of the Obligatory Quality Assurance System was established, as well as the regulation of the IPS and EPS accreditation and accreditation systems.

By means of the Decree of 15 October 2002, compliance was established for Health Service Providers, Health Promotion Entities, Subsidised Regime Administrators, Adapted Entities, Prepaid Medicine Companies and Departmental, District and Municipal Health Entities. In its Article 6, of the

The Decree in question defines the particularities of the SOGC and the SGSSS, with the aim of evaluating and improving the Quality of Health Care, as follows:

- Accessibility. This is the possibility that every user has of being able to enjoy the health services provided by the General Social Security Health System.
- Opportunity. This is the possibility for all users to obtain the services they require without delays that put their lives or health at risk. This factor is related to the organisation of the supply of services in correspondence with demand, and with the degree of institutional coordination to manage access to services.
- Safety. This is constituted as the set of structural elements, processes, instruments and methodologies, based on scientifically proven evidence, that lead to minimising the risk of suffering an adverse event in the health care process or of reducing its consequences.
- Relevance. This is the level at which users obtain the required services, according to scientific evidence, and their marginal effects are minimal to the potential benefits.
- Continuity. This is the level at which users receive the required interventions, through a logical and rational sequence of activities, based on scientific knowledge.

The standard emphasises the need for health organisations to have auditing procedures in place, defines the way they operate and function in each of them EPS, IPS and Territorial Health Directorates (DTS), and also indicates the importance of adopting indicators and standards that help them to specify the expected quality indicators in their care processes. On the basis of this information, these institutions should carry out preventive, follow-up and short-term actions that continuously and systematically measure the ratio between the indicators indicated and the results achieved, in order to fulfil their functions of guaranteeing access, safety, timeliness, relevance and continuity of care and user satisfaction.

Article 40 of this Decree outlines the urgent processes to be evaluated for each of these institutions. For example, both EPSs and ARSs must continue with processes of systematic self-evaluation of the capacity of their health services network, of the implementation of the referral and counter-referral system, as well as checking that all providers in their service network are fully qualified. On the other hand, HPSs are obliged to systematically measure user satisfaction in relation to the fulfilment of their rights, access and timeliness of services.

At the same time, in the IPS the quality audits should focus at least on self-evaluation processes of events identified as urgent, based on the observation of the elements of quality indicated in Decree 1011 of 2006, as well as being able to satisfy users, with in relation to the services offered.

The implementation of the system of qualification for the IPS was regulated by means of Resolution 1043 of 2006, which appropriates the registration forms and new developments for the special registry of health service providers, establishes the manuals of standards and procedures, the situations of patrimonial and financial capacity of the single system of qualification of health service providers.

The Manual of Standards for the Technological and Scientific Conditions of the Unified System of Qualification of Health Service Providers defines the urgent processes that need to be evaluated and monitored by the IPS, as well as the evaluation requirements.

In relation to these processes, it was indicated: Urgent care processes. Standard: The main healthcare processes, internal clinical guidelines or those defined by legal norms are explained. The information contains actions to disseminate their content to the people responsible for their execution and to monitor their performance.

1. Clinical care procedures or guidelines and protocols for health areas are written and prepared, according to the most common procedures in the service, and include activities aimed at confirming their performance.
2. Procedures, processes, guidelines and protocols must be known by the staff in charge and responsible for their execution, including staff in training.
3. The institution maintains clinical care guidelines for those pathologies that make up the first 10 causes of consultation or discharge, officially reported by each of the institution's services such as: hospitalisation, intermediate and intensive care units, burns unit, obstetrics, surgery, outpatient and emergency care.
4. If the institution provides promotion and prevention activities, it must have implemented the technical standards for specific protection and early detection stipulated by health authorities at the national level.

5. The institution follows stipulated procedures for the management of infectious or biohazardous hospital waste.
6. If the institution offering emergency, intensive and intermediate care services has established a procedure for reviewing resuscitation equipment on a shift-by-shift basis; requests for consultation and a structured method of alerting.
7. The institution follows continuous coordination procedures between the infection committee and the sterilisation, cleaning and housekeeping service and hospital maintenance.
8. The institution has guidelines on handling medical gases, changing water tanks and alarm systems.
9. If the institution provides hospital services, especially with intermediate and intensive care units, burn unit, obstetrics, surgery or emergencies, it must have:

- Well-defined procedures for appointment procedures by health and medical areas, and guidelines on the daily medical round of patients' progress.
- Guidelines or manuals for the following procedures: cardio-cerebro-pulmonary resuscitation care, fluid management, health area care plan, medication management, patient immobilisation, venipuncture, laboratory sampling, bladder catheterisation and preparation for diagnostic imaging.

10. If the institution offers intermediate and intensive care unit services, it must have the following in addition to the above:
- Guidelines for feeding tubes, declaration of brain death, intracranial pressure catheter placement, central catheter insertion, transient internal pacemaker insertion, tracheostomy, bronchoscopy, thoracentesis, change of IV lines (central and peripheral), parenteral nutrition monitoring, prophylactic anticoagulation.

General Health Administration Students' Contribution to this Chapter

The implementation of the General Social Security Health System (SGSSS) in Colombia and the emphasis that has been given to the quality of health services provided by Service Providing Institutions (IPS). Several key decrees and regulations related to quality assurance in health care in the country are highlighted, underlining the importance of this aspect in the Colombian health system.

First, Decree 2174 of 1996 established the Obligatory System of Quality Assurance, which was later modified by Decree 2309 of 2002. Then, on 3 April 2006, Decree 1011 of 2006 was issued, which also played a crucial role in regulating quality in health care. In addition, Decree 780 of 2016 consolidated these decrees into the Single Regulatory Decree of the Health and Social

Protection Sector.

The Sistema Obligatorio de Garantía de Calidad de la Atención en Salud (SOGCS) consists of four main elements: the Sistema Único de Habilitación (SUH), the Programa de Auditoría para el Mejoramiento de la Calidad (PAMEC), the Sistema Único de Acreditación (SUA) and the Sistema de Información para la Calidad en Salud (SICS).

In the context of health care in Colombia, it is essential to understand the quality principles set out in Law 100 of 1993. These principles include:

1. **Accessibility:** Ensure that all citizens have the possibility of accessing SGSSS health services.
2. **Timeliness**: Ensuring that required services are available without delays that put the life or health of patients at risk.
3. **Safety**: Implement measures to minimise the risk of adverse events during medical care.
4. **Relevance**: Providing services according to scientific evidence, avoiding unintended marginal effects.
5. **Continuity**: Providing health interventions in a sequential and coherent manner, based on scientific knowledge.

It is relevant to note that Law 100 of 1993 also establishes the obligatory nature of the Quality Assurance Systems and audits that IPS and EPS must follow. The main objective of these systems is to guarantee quality in the provision of health services and to protect the rights to life and health of the Colombian population, as enshrined in the country's Constitution.

In addition, it is mentioned that the National Superintendence of Health issued circulars related to the quality of health care, which demonstrates the importance that the regulatory authorities attach to this aspect.

Analysis

The text elaborates on the relevance of quality of health care in Colombia and highlights the series of regulations and procedures designed to ensure it within the framework of the SGSSS. These measures seek to ensure that Colombian citizens have access to safe, timely and high quality health services.

For the realisation of this, a series of modifications took place which led to the implementation of new decrees and regulations.

Questions What are the quality principles set out in Law 100?

When talking about accessibility, do you think that all citizens have access to quality health services?

This chapter analyses the Hawthorne effect in which studies were carried out to understand how different variables affect employee productivity, with the result that the mere observation of workers during their working day had a significant impact on their performance , as performance improved when they felt observed, affecting quality. but what is quality? The definition of quality has evolved greatly. in the past it was associated with doing things well, regardless of cost or effort. as early as the industrial revolution, quality was referred to as efficient production to satisfy demand and obtain economic benefits, later techniques were implemented to reduce defective products by carrying out so-called quality control, until it evolved to total quality, referring to the satisfaction of customer requirements.

What is quality in health care?

seeks to provide greater benefits with lower risks to the

The perception of quality may vary according to the perspective of the provider, the payer or the user, but the most general definition is to try to meet the needs and expectations of the consumer of health services by breaking down 4 dimensions:

1. Technique: knowledge + equipment.
2. Safety: higher benefits at lower risk.
3. Service: humanised care provided to the user.
4. Cost-benefit ratio: assessing the efficiency and effectiveness of health interventions, enabling the optimal allocation of resources and maximisation of health benefits for the population.

To ensure quality, it is essential to develop quality assurance programmes from individual care to networks of service providers. This implies the implementation of constant measurement and evaluation such as audits, a fundamental tool to evaluate the structure (where health services are provided), the processes (involving specific actions) and the outcomes (benefits obtained).

1) Key finding of the Hawthorne effect.

a. Temperature in the workplace affects productivity.

b. Workers' satisfaction does not influence their performance.

c. Communication and attention from the supervisor can influence productivity.

d. Financial incentives are the main motivation.

2. What is meant by "quality in health care"?

a. Number of patients seen.

b. Availability of advanced technologies in a health centre.

c. Greater benefit with less risk to the user.

d. Doctors' satisfaction with their working conditions.

Chapter 8

Cancer Risk Management Indicators

Cancer is a disease where the patient can do much to help himself if he can maintain his morale and his hopes.

George Carman

Risk Management

Risk is the probability that an event will occur. In Colombia, the Ministry of Health defined risk management as a "strategy to anticipate public health events, diseases and injuries so that they do not occur, or if they do occur, to detect and treat them early in order to mitigate or shorten their evolution or consequences".

According to the WHO, the factors that cause a person to become ill can be spread over several years and influenced by broader socio-economic variables. Education and income levels can influence eating habits and behaviours such as alcohol consumption, which in turn interact with physiological and pathophysiological causes such as blood pressure, cholesterol levels and glucose metabolism to lead to diseases such as stroke and coronary heart disease.

Knowledge of the distribution and determinants of risk is essential for the identification and selection of evidence-based individual and collective interventions aimed at both minimising the risk of disease occurrence and the comprehensive management of the disease when it has occurred.

A risk group is a set of people with common conditions of exposure and vulnerability to certain events who share the natural history of the disease, related risk factors, clinical outcomes and efficient forms or strategies of service delivery.

The risk groups are formed taking into account social risk groups, diseases of high frequency and chronicity, priority diseases in public health, diseases with high-cost treatments, intolerable conditions for society and high-cost diseases. By possessing similar characteristics, it is possible to define an organised and coherent social response established as an integrated sectoral and intersectoral care process that allows for comprehensive management.

The Ten-Year Public Health Plan 2012-2021 conceived health risk as "the probability of the occurrence of an undesirable, avoidable and negative event for the health of the individual, which may also be the worsening of a previous condition or the need to require more consumption of goods and services that could have been avoided". The event is the occurrence of the disease or its unfavourable evolution and its causes are the different associated factors. Health risk can be classified as primary if it refers to the probability of the appearance of new morbidity or its severity, or as technical if it refers to the probability of "the occurrence of events derived from failures of care in health services and the increased burden of disease due to avoidable mortality and disability".

Integrated Health Risk Management

Integrated Health Risk Management (IHRM) is a cross-cutting strategy of the Integrated Health Care Policy, which is based on the articulation and interaction of health system agents and other sectors to identify, evaluate, measure, intervene (from prevention to palliation) and carry out follow-up and monitoring of health risks to individuals, families and communities, aimed at achieving health outcomes and the well-being of the population. ISWM anticipates diseases and injuries so that they do not occur or are detected and treated early to prevent, shorten or mitigate their progression and consequences. The aim of the strategy is to achieve a better level of health of the population, a better user experience during the care process and costs commensurate with the results obtained.

The implementation of the GIRS in a territory is based on the priorities identified in the Territorial Health Plan - PTS, and its intervention through the articulation of population, collective and individual interventions carried out by the agents of the System and other sectors under the coordination of the territorial entity. The Territorial Health Plan is the strategic and indicative instrument of public policy in health, which allows the territorial entities to contribute to the achievement of the strategic goals of the Ten-Year Public Health Plan, in line with the national development plan and the land-use plan, among others.

Risk management programmes emerged in response to scientific advances that allowed the quantification of cancer risk. Once quantified, risk can be reduced through interventions (lifestyle, appropriate treatments, etc.). To provide these benefits to high-risk populations, professionals with specific expertise in these areas are organised into risk management programmes; in the process, cohorts of patients are created for research studies related to cancer risk assessment and prevention.

Over time, risk management programmes have proliferated and expanded in scope, evolving into multidisciplinary bodies that identify women who would benefit from genetic screening, provide recommendations for preventive medication or risk-reducing surgery, help make decisions about the use of advanced screening with magnetic resonance imaging, and recommend lifestyle interventions to reduce risk.

Breast cancer

Breast cancer is the most commonly diagnosed malignancy and the second most common cause of cancer death in women, accounting for about 1 in 10 new cancer diagnoses each year.

In 2019, it was estimated that 30% of women would develop breast cancer in their lifetime and 15% of them would die from it. Incidence, mortality and survival differ significantly between countries and regions. According to Globocan 2020 data, the incidence for breast cancer in Colombia was 15509 new cases, the mortality rate was 4411 and the 5-year prevalence for all ages was 52025 cases.

Breast cancer evolves silently and most disease is discovered in routine screening tests. Survival rates improve with early diagnosis, although the tumour tends to spread lymphatically and haematologically, leading to distant metastases and poor prognosis. Breast cancer screening guidelines increasingly recommend that clinicians perform risk assessment to inform shared decision-making.

From this perspective, precision medicine has become the preferred approach to cancer screening, with the goal of increased surveillance in high-risk women, while avoiding unnecessary imaging burdens in those at lower risk.

Prostate cancer

Prostate cancer is the second most frequent malignant neoplasm (after lung cancer) in men worldwide, with standardised rates x 100,000 of 30.7 for incidence and 7.7 for mortality, representing 3.8% of all deaths caused by cancer in men. In Colombia, it ranks first in both new cases diagnosed and deaths, with rates of 49.8 and 11.9 respectively, and is responsible for a high percentage of cancer deaths in men: 19%. According to the High Cost Account (CAC), by 2020 there were 3692 new cases diagnosed and 2178 deaths.

Both incidence and mortality from this type of cancer worldwide correlates with ageing, with a median age at at diagnosis of 66 years. For black men, incidence rates are higher compared to white men, with 158.3 new cases diagnosed per 100,000 men, and their mortality is approximately twice that of white men.

The reasons for this disparity have been hypothesised on differences in social, environmental and genetic factors. Although 2,293,818 new cases are estimated up to 2040, a small variation in mortality will be observed (an increase of 1.05%).

It is possible that the above increase is due to increased screening for the disease using prostate specific antigen (PSA), which has resulted in declines in mortality in developed countries, but this is not the case in the rest of the world, probably because poverty conditions are a major determinant.

GIRS for breast and prostate cancer

When contextualising risk management within the cancer framework, two moments can be identified:

I Risk before the disease, when healthy people are exposed to the development of cancer due to biological, genetic, social, environmental and lifestyle factors among others, so interventions should focus on these and on specific actions such as performing breast self-examination and screening mammography for early diagnosis in women and prostate antigen testing in men.

2) Risk during the disease: this is referred to when the pathology is established and is related to the possible outcomes: disappearance of the disease, reduction of the disease without disappearing completely, progression when there is no response to treatment, no change in the disease or death.

Interventions need to be more targeted to reduce complications, disease-related disability and ensure quality of life, for which there must be a comprehensive understanding of the clinical aspects.

The risk management indicators for breast and prostate cancer in Colombia defined by High Cost Account are as follows:

Table 3. Risk management indicators for breast cancer in Colombia. 2019

Name	Numerator	Denominator	Range of compliance		
			High	Medium	Under
Proportion of women with breast cancer who underwent TNM staging at NRC.	Number of women with breast cancer who have undergone clinical staging (TNM), CRN	Total number of women diagnosed with breast cancer mum	>90 %	> 80 y < 90%	<80 %
Proportion of women with breast cancer who underwent TNM staging in prevalent.	Number of women with breast cancer who underwent clinical staging (TNM), prevalent	Total number of women diagnosed with breast cancer mum	>90 %	> 80 y < 90%	<80 %
Proportion of women with breast cancer detected as as carcinomas in situ at diagnosis.	Number of women detected as carcinomas in situ at diagnosis	Total number of women diagnosed with breast cancer mum	> 12 %	>6y < 12 %	< 6 %
Proportion of women with breast cancer detected in stages early at the time of diagnosis.	Number of women detected as early stage invasive carcinomas at the time of diagnosis	Total number of women diagnosed with invasive breast cancer	>50 %	> 42 y < 50%	<42 %

Proportion of women with breast cancer detected at advanced stages at diagnosis.	Number of women detected as advanced stage invasive carcinomas at the time of diagnosis	Total number of women diagnosed with invasive breast cancer	<50 %	< 57 y > 50%	>58 %
Proportion of patients with diagnosis histopathology prior to surgery.	Number of women with histopathological diagnosis before surgery	Total number of women who can be found at underwent surgery	>70 %	> 40 y < 70%	<40 %
Proportion of women with breast cancer with a hormone receptor (oestrogen/progesterone) finding	Number of women with breast cancer with hormone receptor (oestrogen/progesterone) result	Total number of women who can be found at underwent surgery	>90 %	>70 y < 90%	<70 %
Proportion of patients with HER2 study.	Number of women with invasive breast cancer with HER2 status result	Total women diagnosed	>90 %	>70 y < 90%	<70 %

Name	**Numerator**	**Denominator**	**Range of compliance**		
			High	**Medium**	**Under**
		with invasive breast cancer			
Proportion of women with invasive breast cancer who have undergone	Number of patients with invasive breast cancer who underwent breast-conserving surgery	Total from patients with invasive	>90 %	>70 y < 90%	<70 %

Name	Numerator	Denominator	Range of compliance		
			High	Medium	Under
surgery surgery the breast.		breast cancer who received treatment surgical			
Proportion of women with in situ breast cancer who underwent surgery surgery breast conservation.	Number of patients with in situ breast cancer who underwent breast-conserving surgery	Total from patients with in situ breast cancer who were treated surgically	>70 %	> 50 y < 70%	50 %
Proportion of breast cancer patients who underwent radiotherapy after breast cancer treatment.	Number of breast cancer patients who underwent radiotherapy after breast-conserving surgery	Total from breast cancer patients who have been diagnosed with	>90 %	>70 y < 90%	<70 %
breast conserving surgery (CNR)		performed breast-conserving surgery			
Proportion of women with r ecipients hormone-positive women who are given hormone blockade as a treatment.	Number of women with hormone receptor-positive invasive breast cancer receiving hormone blockade treatment	Total women with invasive breast cancer and positive hormone receptors	>90 %	> 80 y < 90%	<80 %
Proportion of	Number of women with	Total	>70	>34,1 y	34,1

women who received anti-HER2 therapy.	invasive breast cancer who received anti-HER2 therapy	number of women with invasive breast cancer with HER2 receptor (+)	%	< 70 %	%
Timeliness of overall care (time between consultation for presence of cancer-associated symptoms to first treatment).	Sum of days between referral note from general practitioner/institution to diagnosing institution and first treatment for women with breast cancer (includes in situ).	Total women with breast cancer (including in situ)	<60 days	<75y> 60 days	>75 days

Name	**Numerator**	**Denominator**	**Range of compliance**		
			High	**Medium**	**Under**
Timeliness of cancer care (time between between the diagnosis until the first treatment).	Sum of days between diagnosis and first treatment for women with breast cancer (includes in situ)	Total women with breast cancer (including in situ)	<30 days	< 45 and > 30 days	>45 days
Timeliness of care by the treating physician (time between valid histopathological report and care by the treating physician).	Sum of days between valid histopathological report and care by treating physician for women with breast cancer (including in situ).	Total women with breast cancer (including in situ)	< 15 days	<30 y >15 days	>30 days
Timeliness of treatment initiation (time between care by	Sum of days between care by treating physician and start of first treatment (surgery, chemotherapy,	Total women with breast cancer (including in	< 15 days	< 30 and > 15 days	>30 days

treating physician to first treatment).	radiotherapy, hormone blockade, palliative care) (days), for women with breast cancer (including in situ)	situ)			
Name	**Numerator**	**Denominator**	**Range of compliance**		
			High	**Medium**	**Under**
Timeliness of initiation of adjuvant therapy (time from surgery to first treatment) treatment post-surgical: radiotherapy/hormone blockade).	Sum of the days between surgery and the first post-surgical treatment (chemotherapy/radiotherapy/hormone blockade) (days), in women with breast cancer (excludes in situ)	Total women with breast cancer (excludes in situ)	<42 days	< 56 and > 42 days	>56 days
Breast cancer case fatality (stages early)	Number of women with breast cancer who died during the period (by stage: Early stages)	Total number of women with breast cancer during the period (according to stage: 1,000, 1,000, 1,000, 1,000, 1,000, 1,000) stage: early)	<1, 3 %	<2y> 1,3 %	≥
Breast cancer	Number of women with breast	Total	<4,	<5y>	5%

case fatality (stages advanced)	cancer who died during the period (by stage: Advanced Stages)	number of women with breast cancer during the period (according to stage: 1,000, 1,000, 1,000, 1,000, 1,000, 1,000) st age: advanced)	4 %	4,4 %	

Source: High Cost Account, 2022

Table 4. Risk management indicators for prostate cancer in Colombia, 2019

Indicator Name	Numerator	Denominator	Cut-off points
1. Timeliness of diagnosis in days; time between the consultation where a referral is made for clinical or paraclinical suspicion associated with prostate cancer until diagnosis.	Sum of the difference in days between referral on suspicion and diagnosis, valid in the reporting period.	Total number of diagnosed patients with valid dates in the reporting period.	<30 days >=30-60days >=60 days
2. Proportion of patients with TNM-staged prostate cancer	Number of incident patients with prostate cancer staged by TNM at the time of d.	Total incident patients diagnosed with prostate cancer.	>90% >60-<=90% <=60 %
3. Proportion of patients with localised prostate cancer (stage 0,1 and II patients).	Patients with prostate cancer TNM stages O+I+II	Total number of patients staged at all TNM stages	>69% >62-<=69% <=62 %
4. Proportion of patients with locally advanced prostate cancer y advanc ed (stage III and IV patients).	Patients with prostate cancer TNM stage III+IV	Total number of patients staged at all TNM stages.	<31% >31-<=37% >=37 %
5. Proportion of staged patients with Gleason score.	Number of incident patients with breast cancer	Total number of incident patients reported	>90% >85 - <=90% <=85 %
Indicator Name	**Numerator**	**Denominator**	**Cut-off points**
	prostate who had undergone Gleason staging	histopathological y CIEC6IX0D.	
6. Timeliness of	Incident sum of the	Total number of	<30 days

treatment in days, time from diagnosis to first treatment.	difference in days between histopathological report and first treatment.	incident patients diagnosed in treatment with valid dates.	>=30-<60 days >=60 days

Source: High Cost Account, 2022

Analysis of risk management indicators for cancer in Colombia

Based on the information in the High Cost Account, which is open access, through free registration on the SISCAC platform, the information necessary for the development of this analysis was taken.

Breast Cancer

Figura 11. Proportion of reported new cases of breast cancer with TNM staging, at the

TNM staging, nationally and by department in Colombia, 2023.

departments in Colombia, 2023

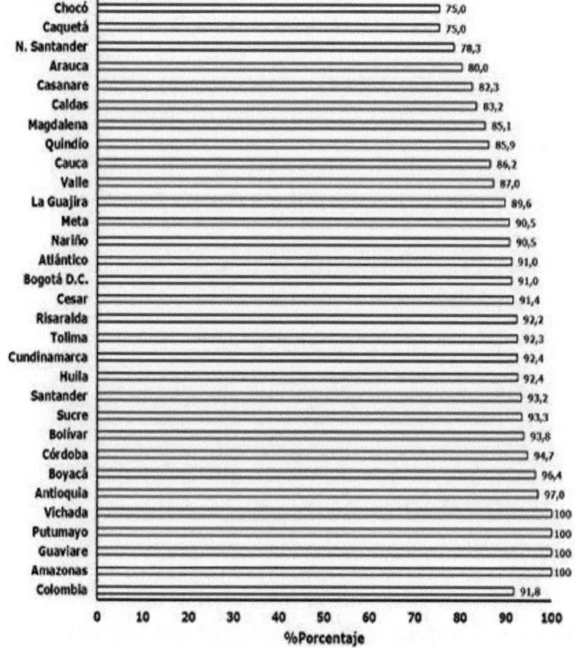

Fuente: CAC, 2023

The proportion of women with breast cancer who underwent TNM staging in NRC (New Cases Reported) at the national level was 91.8%. Three departments had values considered as "low compliance": Norte de Santander, Caquetá and Chocó; the rest had medium or high compliance (Figure 11).

Figura 12. Proportion of women with breast cancer who underwent TNM staging in prevalent
TNM staging in prevalent breast cancer, nationally and by department in departments in Colombia, 2022

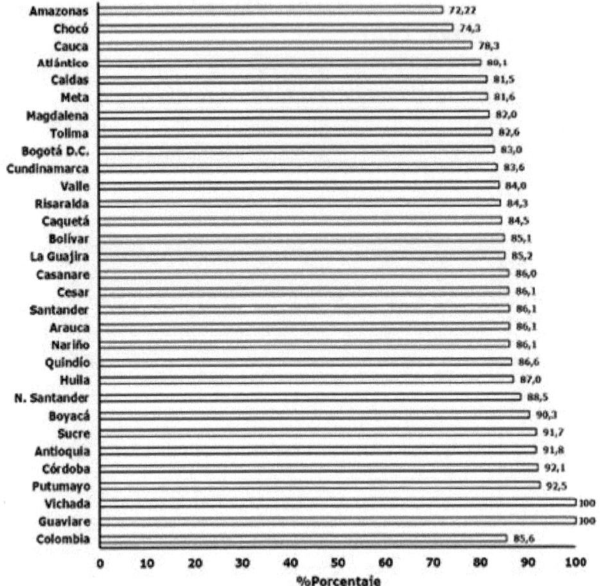

Source: ACC, 2023

Only eight departments had values considered high: Guainía, Guaviare, Vichada, Putumayo, Córdoba, Antioquia, Sucre and Boyacá, and at the other extreme, three had low values: Cauca, Chocó and Amazonas (Figure 12).

Figura 13. Proportion of women with breast cancer detected at advanced stages at the time of diagnosis
at diagnosis, nationally and by department in Colombia, 2022.
departments in Colombia, 2022

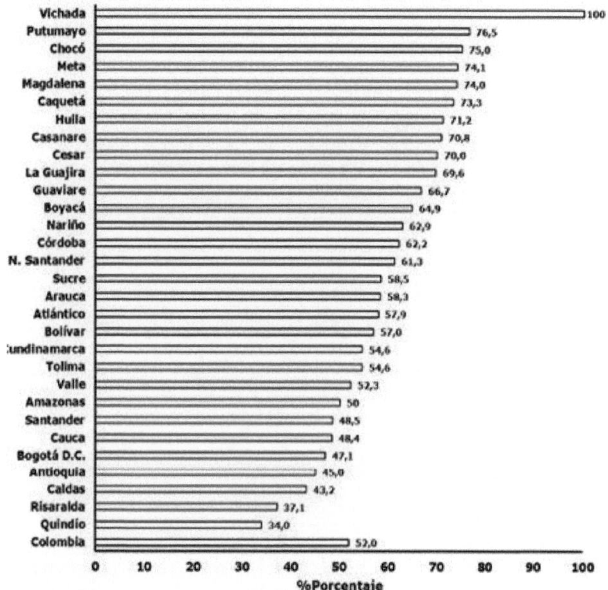

Source: ACC, 2023

52% of patients with TNM staging are diagnosed at advanced stages, a value considered high by CAC; in fact, the vast majority of departments showed a negative aspect in this indicator by having high percentages of detection at advanced stages, with Vichada, Putumayo and Chocó being the most severe cases (Figure 13).

Figura 14. Overall timeliness of care, nationally and by department in Colombia, 2022
departments in Colombia, 2022

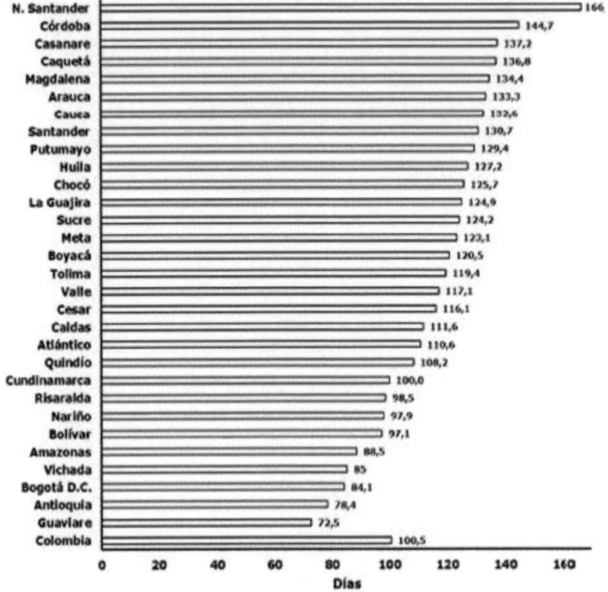

Fuente: CAC, 2023

The overall timeliness of care, i.e. the time between consultation for the presence of symptoms associated with cancer until the first treatment, showed extremely worrying values for the country, as the average was 100.5 days at the national level and all departments had times of more than 70 days, with Norte de Santander being of high concern with 166.5 days (Figure 14).

Figura 15. Early-stage breast cancer case fatality, nationally and by department in
nationally and by department in Colombia, 2022

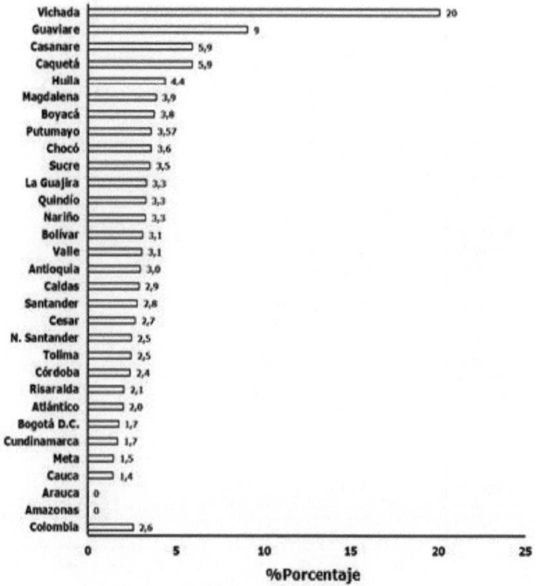

Fuente: CAC, 2023

The early stage case fatality rate in Colombia was 2.6%; most departments had values below 6%, but Vichada had an alarming 20% (Figure 15).

Prostate

Figure 16. Prostate cancer diagnosis opportunity at national level and by department in 2022

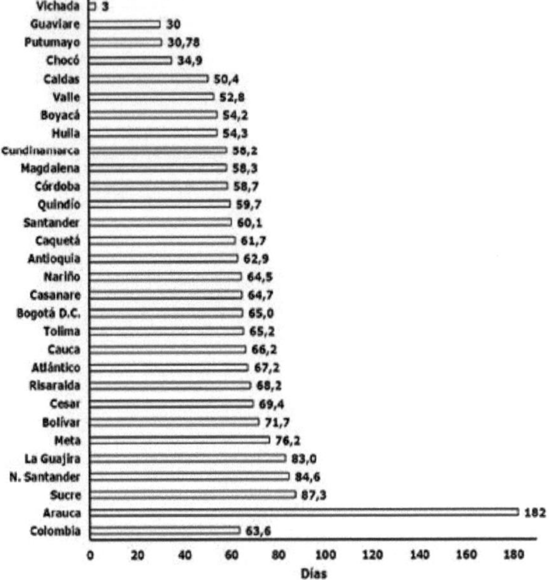

Fuente: CAC, 2023

The national diagnostic timeliness was 63.6 days. Fourteen departments were above this value, with Arauca being significantly higher (182) (Figure 16).

Figure 17. Percentage of prostate cancer patients staged by TNM nationally and by department in 2022

TNM at the national level and by department in 2022

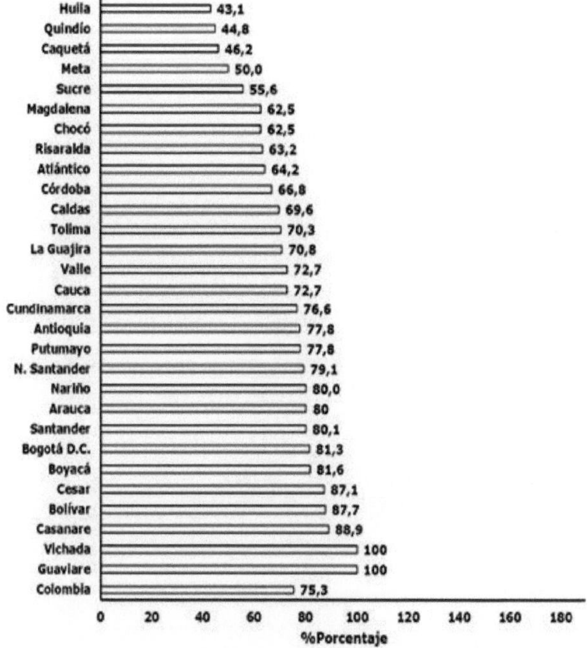

Nationally, only 75.3% of patients are staged. Sixteen departments are below this value, with figures ranging from 72.7% for Cauca to 43.1% in Huila (Figure 17).

Figure 18. Opportunity of treatment of prostate cancer patients, nationally and by department in 2022

Figura 18. Oportunidad de tratamiento de pacientes con cáncer de próstata, a nivel nacional y por departamentos en 2022

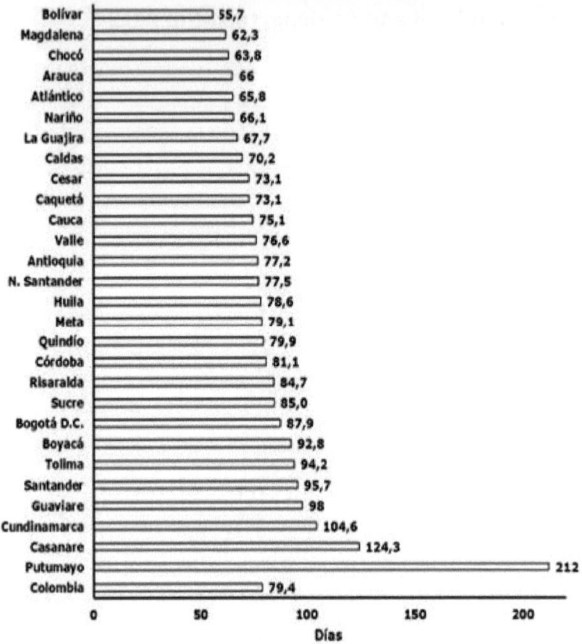

Fuente: CAC, 2023

The national timeliness of treatment was 79.4 days. Eleven departments were above this value, with Putumayo being the most notorious, with 212 days (Figure 18).

CONCLUSION

Early detection of prostate cancer decreases mortality, an important indicator as indicated in a study, where the national average for timeliness of diagnosis was 62.5 days. However, this value is far from ideal, since the opportunity in terms of time to access health services should be guaranteed for individuals, especially in pathologies that affect the quality of life, the economy and the optimal functioning of the individual in society and according to CAC, the optimal value of this indicator should be less than 30 days, a figure that was not achieved by most of the departments.

Diagnostic and treatment opportunities show worrying values, as they are likely to be associated with a higher case fatality rate in advanced stages.

General Health Administration Students' Contribution to this Chapter with

Risk Management.

Considering that risk is the probability of an event occurring, **risk management** is a strategy to anticipate in public health, to mitigate or shorten the evolution of diseases and their consequences.

In this sense, it is important to know the determinants of risk in order to determine interventions aimed at minimising the risk of disease occurrence and, if it has already occurred, to determine how to manage it.

Risk groups.

These are groups of people with common conditions of vulnerability; history of the disease, risk factors. They are formed according to:

- Highly chronic diseases
- Diseases of high public health priority.
- Diseases with high-cost treatments.

In this way it is possible to define an organised social proposal for the integral care process.

Primary risk. Occurrence of a new morbidity or its severity.

Technical risk. Probability of occurrence of events due to failures in health care services and of increased burden of disease due to avoidable morbidity or mortality and disability.

Breast cancer. It is the most common diagnosis and the second most common cause of cancer death in women. It evolves silently, the survival rate improves with early diagnosis, so physicians should make a risk assessment to inform decision making.

Prostate cancer. It is the second most frequent diagnosis in men worldwide (after lung cancer). In Colombia, it ranks first in both new diagnoses and deaths.

Both incidence and mortality, worldwide, correlate with ageing (mean age at diagnosis, 66 years). For black men the incidence is higher compared to white men.

Integrated Health Risk Management (IHRM)

It is a transversal strategy of the integrated health care policy, based on the articulation and interaction of the agents of the health system and other sectors to identify, evaluate, measure (from prevention to palliation) and carry out follow-up and monitoring of health risks for all. It anticipates diseases and injuries so that they do not occur or are detected and treated to prevent their evolution and consequences.

The objective of this strategy is to achieve a better level of health for the population. The implementation of ISWM in a territory is based on the priorities identified in the Territorial Health Plan, which is the instrument that allows territorial entities to contribute to the achievement of the strategic goals of the ten-year public health plan and the national development plan, among others.

Risk management programmes emerged in response to scientific advances that enabled the quantification of cancer. Over time, risk management programmes have broadened their scope and evolved.

Placing risk management in the cancer framework identifies two moments:

1. Risk before the disease: healthy people exposed to developing cancer due to different factors; biological, genetic, social, environmental, lifestyles, among others.

Prevention focuses on breast self-examination, screening mammograms and prostate antigen screening in men.

2. Risk during the disease: the pathology is already established and is related to the possible outcomes; disappearance of the disease, decrease of the disease, progression, no change or death.

Cancer risk management in Colombia is assessed by indicators. The evaluation of the indicators has a range of compliance classified as high, medium and low; there are 14 indicators for breast cancer and 6 for prostate cancer.

Examples:

Indicator:

proportion of women with breast cancer who underwent TNM stabilisation at CNR.

Result:

The following were considered to have medium compliance: sucre, la guajira, choco, atlántico, Magdalena and meta, the rest had high compliance.

Indicator:

Proportion of patients with TNM-staged prostate cancer.

Result:

Nationally only 72.4% of patients are staged, 13 patients are below this value with figures ranging from 68.8% for Nariño to 33.3% for Casanare.

Suggestions.

From our point of view, the development and approach to the subject matter is adequate and easy to understand . However, we consider it necessary to add a glossary describing the meaning of the acronyms mentioned throughout the chapter, as this would make it even easier to understand, especially for those who are not familiar with the subject.

Finally, we would like to state that, during the reading and analysis, we questioned ourselves about the location of the chapter within the book and we came to the conclusion that the theme developed in it does not have the expected relationship with the themes that have been dealt with up to that point and the following ones, so we believe that it would be better placed at the end of the book.

Questions:

1. What is the objective of health risk management?

a) Mitigate or shorten the progression of diseases.

b) Mitigate or shorten the consequences of diseases.

c) a and b are true.

d) None of the above.

2. How is public health risk classified?

a) Primary risk and secondary risk.

b) Primary risk, secondary risk and tertiary risk.

c) Primary risk and technical risk.

d) None of the above.

3. What characteristics are taken into account to form risk groups?

a) High-cost treatments

b) Highly chronic diseases

c) Priority diseases in public health.

d) All of the above.

4. is the objective of the ISWM strategy?

a) The articulation and interaction of health actors.

b) Identify, assess, measure, intervene, follow up and monitor health risks.

c) Achieving a better level of population health, a better user experience during the care process and costs commensurate with the results obtained.

d) None of the above.

5. Why did risk management programmes emerge?

a) They arose to treat illness and trauma.

b) They arose to ensure the quality of life

c) They arose in response to scientific advances that allowed the quantification of cancer.

d) None of the above.

Risk Management.

Considering that risk is the probability of an event occurring, risk management is a strategy to anticipate in public health, to mitigate or shorten the evolution of diseases and their consequences.

In this sense, it is important to know the determinants of risk in order to determine interventions aimed at minimising the risk of disease occurrence and, if it has already occurred, to determine how to manage it.

Risk groups.

These are groups of people with common conditions of vulnerability; history of the disease, risk factors. They are formed according to:

- Highly chronic diseases
- Diseases of high public health priority.
- Diseases with high-cost treatments.

In this way it is possible to define an organised social proposal for the integral care process.

Primary risk. Occurrence of a new morbidity or its severity.

Technical risk. Probability of occurrence of events due to failures in health care services and of increased burden of disease due to avoidable morbidity and disability.

Breast cancer. It is the most common diagnosis and the second most common cause of cancer death in women. It evolves silently, the survival rate improves with early diagnosis, so physicians should make a risk assessment to inform decision making.

Prostate cancer. It is the second most frequent diagnosis in men worldwide (after lung cancer). In Colombia, it ranks first in both new diagnoses and deaths.

Both incidence and mortality, worldwide, correlate with ageing (mean age at diagnosis, 66 years). For black men the incidence is higher compared to white men.

Health management and its use in my professional life.

Health administration or health administration is the social and technical science related to the planning, organisation, management and control of public and private enterprises in the health sector, through the optimisation of financial, technological and human resources.

Chapter 9

Predictive Health

Sometimes when you innovate, you make mistakes. It's better to admit them quickly, and move on to your other innovations", Steve Jobs.

Underlying all treatment is the principle "Primum Non Nocere", which can be considered as a basic principle in health care delivery activity that should focus first on doing no harm. Despite this, and due to the complexity of treatment, the individual component of a person interacts with various factors. The structure, tasks or procedures of the patient's physical environment, including material, technical equipment and the physical place where care is provided or organised, are sometimes the cause of adverse events that may occur more frequently than recommended. Recent technological advances have brought about great changes in society, allowing complex situations to be identified and acted upon in a timely manner.

Table 5. Main points of predictive medicine

Predictive medicine
- .. Predicting an individual's response to a treatment
- To guess which people are at risk for a certain disease, either because of genetic load, family history or lifestyle habits.
- Predicting the evolution of a patient suffering from a disease.
- Anticipation that allows planning prevention strategies, early initiation of treatment, better prognosis.
J.M. Piqué. Med. Clin.2013; 140(11): 514-519

The Public Health Emergency of International Concern (PHEIC) caused by COVID-19 has prompted countries to improve their capacities
functional systems, in particular those related to emergency coordination, collaborative surveillance, clinical care and risk communication and communication engagement. Following the pandemic generated by zoonotic transmission of the coronavirus, preparedness systems need to be strengthened: to succeed in identifying, anticipating and detecting the emergence of potentially pandemic pathogens based on a "One Health" approach integrating animal and human health; build essential public health capacities and mobilise personnel for surveillance, early detection and dissemination of information on outbreaks and similar events; strengthen health systems based on universal health coverage and ensure that they have the capacity to cope with a surge in demand for clinical and support services ; and put in place social protection systems to safeguard the vulnerable and leave no one behind.

Following the lessons learned from the COVID-19 pandemic, health systems require ongoing preparedness for an outbreak response of epidemic concern with strategies for rapid and timely exchange of relevant pathogen, sample and genetic sequence information to assist in public health surveillance and response, including identification of effective countermeasures; regulations for the world to have equal access to information on these and other regulations; to rapidly deploy WHO teams for investigation and rapid response; to maintain global supply chains; and to prevent zoonotic risks. Annual active multi-sectoral simulation exercises are highly recommended to continuously assess risks and follow-up measures for mitigation, transnational learning and accountability, and to establish independent, impartial and regular evaluation mechanisms.

In this context, the concept of predictive medicine, which began to develop from knowledge of the histocompatibility system, is gaining momentum with the findings of genomic medicine. Predictive medicine can be considered as the identification of possible diseases to be suffered by healthy individuals. Disease management is evolving towards a more personal and individualised approach as more data on clinical, biochemical, radiological, molecular, histopathological and genetic aspects become available.

Predictive analytics has become the centrepiece of any healthcare analytics strategy. It is now an essential tool for measuring, aggregating and understanding behavioural, psychosocial and biometric data that until recently was either unavailable or extremely difficult to capture. At the individual level, predictive analytics can help healthcare institutions deliver the right care, to the right patient, at the right time. Similarly, it can enable health systems to identify and understand larger trends, leading to public health strategies.

Predictive medicine also makes it possible to identify individuals who do not have a certain predisposition or who are even protected by a specific genetic resistance. Thus, the goal of predictive medicine is to identify susceptibility or resistance to certain diseases in the healthy individual. A major paradigm shift from a corrective to a predictive situation, anticipating the facts, using all available technology to prevent the occurrence of events that affect individual or collective health. Advances in the field of health diagnostics are making it possible to predict and anticipate disease behaviour. Unlike many preventive interventions that target groups, predictive medicine is done on an individualised basis.

While it is true that primary health care is a step that should be prioritised, it is not sufficient to reach the total health coverage of the population, nor can it be able to indicate which pathologies could over time become a burden for the state.

Many health systems focus too little on prevention to focus solely on the curative model, i.e. waiting for people to present with their pathologies before medical care can be provided, so that diseases can only be considered to be cured once they appear on the horizon.

The predictive model is the opposite, pathologies are not expected to occur, but can be foreseen and anticipated so that they do not become public health problems.

In order to implement this model, it is necessary to have all the resources, and it is the State that must provide the vast majority of them, such as a communications infrastructure that reaches all corners of the territory, as the Internet is the ideal means of communication, and through this network, networks of health professionals can be established who are able to study the different cases in order to issue concepts that will determine which could potentially become health risks, and with this knowledge disseminate it to the rest of the territory, which could prevent health and economic losses due to not considering them in a timely manner.

The predictive model in public health must be based first and foremost on epidemiological surveillance, making use of all the technological tools at its disposal in order to know in advance the sequence of cases that, through detailed research, will eventually become chronic pathologies that will require the country's scarce resources, which can be invested in other economic aspects.

Realising this new way of implementing health delivery would welcome a predictive health model in which the social determinants of health are prioritised.

In order to develop a predictive public health model, it is necessary:

Be able to proactively, meaningfully and qualitatively identify conditions at group, household and individual levels that may threaten the health and well-being of residents, families and individuals, and be able to work across sectors to overcome, reduce and transform. in the context of overcoming inequality. Help maintain a centralised information system managed by all health actors and a continuous health screening, research and monitoring system to predict developmental, behavioural and socio-epidemiological parameters in all regions. Planning and capacity to carry out appropriate and accurate promotion and prevention activities at the collective, family and individual levels.

Chapter 10

Health Administration

Success in management requires learning as fast as the world is changing.
Warren Bennis

Health management is a part of general management science that introduces the concepts of planning, organising, directing and controlling organisations to achieve the goals of organisational efficiency and effectiveness by optimising the necessary financial, technical and human resources. The vision of population health management involves addressing the determinants of health. In contrast to personalised care, which focuses on the clinical risks and factors associated with specific diseases. The PLECOSER method has been used for population-wide continuous health improvement processes.

The functional management of the health services market and its facilitated analysis is based on the assumption that health services are developed by service providers who develop products using labour, supply and technology to promote, prevent, diagnose, treat and rehabilitate a specific disease, thereby improving people's well-being and quality of life.

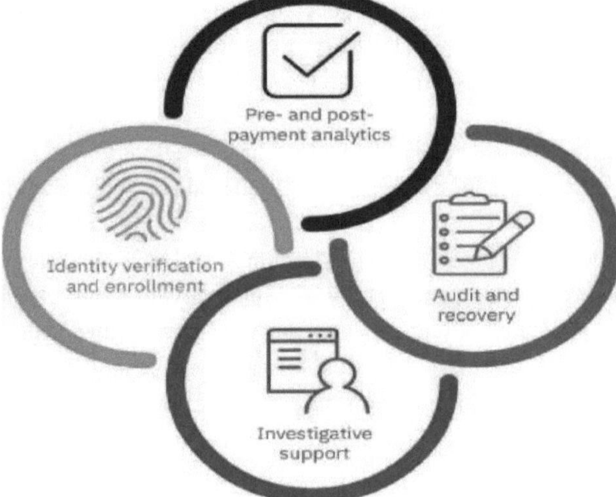

Figure 19. Functional management in the service model

Based on these principles, it is necessary to consider in a general way that the main objectives of healthcare management are to improve, maintain and minimise management risks. The first phase of implementation of a shared model of healthcare management requires that organisational partners are part of the process so that they can commit to the vision and mission of the organisation and thus benefit from a true transformation of healthcare management. Having done this, it is important to plan, to make an outline of the processes that are executed by area, where the whole path is added, even the easiest steps should be described. In summary, health management is a complex and multidisciplinary discipline that seeks to improve efficiency and effectiveness in the delivery of health services. Through the application of administrative principles, health managers contribute to ensuring quality, sustainable and patient-centred health care.

In order to have an adequate approach to assess the capacity of health services to satisfy the needs and their provision to the population, it is necessary to determine how the supply and demand of health services is established, starting from the establishment of a sequence of goods and services produced by a unit of production by certain health service providers. From this flow, patients require these goods and services in order to improve their health condition and thus their quality of life, which is why health is understood as an indispensable good for society, which is why it is the state that must be in charge of normalising the essential figures in order to meet the needs in the context of the setting as a public good.

In addressing this issue, it is important to refer to the behaviour of the different actors that are part of the health market. In the first place, there are the users, who understand not only the people but also the products of health goods and services that are an integral part of the care process.

It should be borne in mind that the provision of health services is offered by the IPS, regardless of their legal nature. These companies or institutions have the productive resources, understood in financial terms; income, buildings and technology, as well as the human talent, which are organised in terms of time of use or working hours reserved to carry out the health care work.

In order to provide health services, it is necessary to mix a set of elements called factors and use them in the best possible way, which is called the productive function. The raw materials to be taken into account for the provision of health services are work, understood as the total hours offered by the personnel or human talent in health, only considering the health care part, and within the capital there must be physical capital, which is understood as the buildings, instruments and inputs, in addition to the human talent, or the skills that must be considered together with the human talent in health.

The goods and services produced and offered in the health market do not only fulfil the role of minimising costs, but also interact with an existing demand, and thus their efficiency will have to be evaluated, among other things, primarily by their close relationship to being able to meet the health requirements of a population.

Within the description of the contexts and particularities of the requirements for health services, the intervention of regulatory factors and possible generations of intervention in pricing and the form of presentation of the goods and services to be provided is assumed. It is necessary to start from the consideration of the individual, willing to consume with the aim of maximising his or her benefit. It is necessary to devise a strategy with a sense of family and community orientation where integrated management can be implemented in individual and group care, in order to plan, implement and control community actions, in a context with a vision of family and community health which has to be driven by the primary provider.

On the other hand, it is necessary to keep in mind the public health management processes that the primary provider executes, such as: (i) cooperation between the different sectors related to the interaction with socio-health services; (ii) knowledge management in terms of training on early detection, concrete protection, analysis, restitution, repair and corrective care, both in the management of human talent and in the processes and procedures to be carried out.

It must be understood that the public offer of health services is oriented towards the identification of a professionalisation of the providers in primary providers on a broad scale, and the offer that is currently available with important technological requirements is considered as complementary providers and in this way the objective of the provision of health services is achieved, in the population with its particularities, demands and possibilities in health, and in this way it is possible to guarantee an offer of health services that is attuned to its situations and conveniences, which allows to achieve the results of health and wellbeing.

The determination of the demand for health services is composed as the sum of indicated population subgroups with certain characteristics, but intertwined with a crucial factor tending to minimise the risk of contracting disease or the comprehensive management of the disease in the short, medium or long term so that no negative effects are produced in the person. The allusion to the particular concept of demand determination for the advances incorporated in the Methodology arises from the analyses and modelling that have been evolving by researchers such as Aday and Andersen (1995), where it has been established that the shift in focus from models of health service utilisation with an element of analysis from the family to the individual is directed especially at the problem of implementing measures at the family level where the diversity of family members is taken into account as a summary indicator of the "family health status".

The conformation and organisation of the health services authorised to provide health services and technologies of both an individual and collective nature, with a tendency towards the solution of the most frequent events, but with the lowest technological requirements, according to the regulations published by the Ministry of Health and Social Protection. The primary part of the network, in spite of its conformation and structuring, is subordinated to carrying out the primary health activities requested by the population to be covered according to its health status and must be able to support the development of activities related to integral risk management, family and community health, primary health care, the differential approach and health care.

In the Comprehensive Registers of Health Service Providers (RIPSS), the primary element emphasises the "resolution of the most frequent events, at the personal, family and community level, during all moments of the life course and in the different settings", while the additional element is responsible for "the individual actions of greater complexity in care, for which they use the referral from the primary component and its counter-referral to it, to guarantee the comprehensiveness and continuity of care".

In this sense, the primary element is considered the structuring support of the RIPSS to provide comprehensive health care for the most relevant events or requests for activities and procedures in accordance with the needs of the population affiliated to the EPS, as well as education and promotion, prevention, comprehensive health risk management and monitoring of compliance and safety of the comprehensive health care routes. To this end, it is necessary to bear in mind, among other things: (i) the Department or District where the EPS is accredited to operate, and therefore the identification and parameterisation of the population affiliated to the EPS, (ii) the provision, suitability and completeness of the health services offer established for that element bearing in mind the characteristics of the population's demand for health services and the defined geographical environment and (iii) the components and instruments according to the planning and specifically designed for the administration for the provision of health services, as stipulated by the Comprehensive Health Care Policy, for health care and comprehensive health risk management and comprehensive health care pathways for fully identified risk groups.

Questionnaire

1. What are the stages of the PLECOSER method used for continuous improvement in health?
2. What is the functional management of the health services market based on?
3. What factors determine the demand for health services?

4. How is the public provision of health services oriented?
5. What is the importance of cooperation between different sectors in public health administration?

Chapter 11

Health Audit

We always have a lot to learn in health Anonymous

Undoubtedly, the improvement of the quality of patient care has reached a significant evolution in recent times, becoming a key element for an accurate diagnosis and treatment, giving rise to the professionalisation of Medical Auditing as a specialisation within the practice of medicine.

The methodical study of the health care process supported by the medical record, its examination and evaluation against diagnostic and treatment protocols, always bearing in mind evidence-based medicine, allows medical auditing to be treated as an essential speciality for health care institutions.

The health audit becomes an important part of the evaluation of processes and the development of strategies for continuous improvement in health systems. It is a methodically developed evaluation system, which has all the means for analysis that can guide towards the scoring and improvement of care processes. It is the branch of medicine that performs the methodical and objective review of the organisation of professional work and medical care, in other words, clinical auditing.

The identification of quality in health presents different possible points of view, it is not only a matter of having to comply with a medical prescription. There are many conditions that come into play, such as the bioavailability and pharmacokinetics of a generic medicine, situations that do not directly involve the doctor, but which are notoriously compromising in the study of results. The doctor-patient relationship marked by the concept of care by making the relationship impersonal, preventing the detection of many psychosomatic symptoms.

BACKGROUND

The first reference is found in Hammurabi's Code of Laws in 1750 B.C., where a writing in ancient Babylonian appears inscribed on a diorite footprint apparently about three metres high; on its upper part, Hammurabi can be seen in relief receiving the laws from the god Samash, which was discovered in Iran and was later transferred to the Louvre Museum in Paris. It accepts the penalty of Talion, the famous law of "an eye for an eye and a tooth for a tooth", and severely punishes negligence.

One of the great guidelines of medicine has been the *Hippocratic oath* dating back to 460 B.C., which explicitly states in one of its sections that "... no one who does not know how to do it shall practice bladder carving", pointing precisely to a topic of quality that, despite the passage of time, has not been conceptualised in its true dimension.

By the 19th century on the Black Sea peninsula, during the Crimean War in 1854 when the nations of England and France invaded the peninsula on the northern coast to favour Turkey in its war against Russia, following the initial success at the Battle of Alma River, there was an unparalleled death toll in British hospitals. By January 1855, there were 3168 deaths: 83 from wounds, 2761 from infectious diseases and 300 from unspecified causes. Because of this situation, the British parliament empowered Nurse Florence Nightingale to report to the hospitals at Scutari near Constantinople. The story about the Barrack Hospital is frightening, it was flooded with sewage and there was no supply of drinking water, inferring the conditions of that facility. After analysing the situation, he proposed to solve it in the short term.

The case of the Scutari hospital is a pioneering report on the quality of medical care and possible solutions, and it is important to underline that in Scutari the mortality rate dropped from 40% of soldiers admitted to hospital to 2% in the following six months.

In 1910, Dr. Emory Codman in Boston, Massachusetts, conducted a retrospective investigation of surgical interventions after the year of their performance.

By 1914 Ernest Codman, chairman of the Hospital Standardisation Committee of the American College of Surgeons, at that time stated as "the objective of the evaluation of better quality medicine" and, in addition, the recognition and grading of hospitals in the United States.

In 1918 the American College of Surgeons (ACS - U.S.A.) establishes the basis for hospital organic conformation and the minimum guidelines for achieving accreditation.

During 1927, Gustav Ward, who carried out an investigation of postoperative mortality and infection for each surgeon, published his results of 8 years of work in New York Women's Hospitals comparing rates. It turned out to be a supposedly effective method.

By 1928 Tomás Pontón, taught a plan for accounting for professional services. Today, the *Medical Audit* is one of the important elements in qualifying and recognising hospitals in the United States and other countries.

In 1950 the University of Michigan conducted a pilot study in 15 hospitals, and after two years of implementation by the medical staff, it was institutionalised .

By 1955 Virgil N. Slee, publicises the procedure as a resource for Continuing Medical Education to reduce morbidity.

In 1963, the medical audit is used in 281 hospitals in 41 US states, greatly expanding the initial coverage of the 15 institutions in 1950, with hospitals of up to 975 beds.

During 1980 the previous experience is expanded to all modern hospitals, based on simple procedures that become standardised with satisfactory results.

The revolution in medical education at the beginning of the 20th century occurred at the same time as a measurement of the quality of care. Abraham Flexner in 1910 in a report for the Carniege Foundation literally stated that he saw "wretched hospitals, death traps without sufficient equipment to perform an ordinary clinical examination" and led the American College of Surgeons to impose minimum standards for the profession and the teaching of medicine became the sole preserve of the universities.

In 1972, the Professional Standards Review Organisation (PSRO) Act was passed in the United States.

In Britain in 1967 the Cogwheel report on maternal mortality and the Hospital Advisory Service (HAS) in 1969 were the initial efforts to audit, however, the paper *Working for Patients* was a breakthrough in the evolution of Medical Audit.

In Colombia, the legal norms that refer to health auditing are as follows:

- Law 100 Title 4 Article 227
- Decree 1570 of 1994
- Decree 1486 of 1994
- Resolution 3905 of 1994
- Resolution 0320 of 1997
- Resolution 04252 of 1997
- Decree 1011 of 2006
- Resolutions 1043 of 2006
- Resolutions 1445 of 2006
- Resolutions 1446 of 2006

Auditing for Quality Improvement in Health Care.

It is defined as the methodical and continuous mechanism of evaluation and improvement of quality compared to the expected quality of health care achieved by users.

The audit programmes implemented in the institutions must be in line with the internationality of the accreditation standards and better than those indicated as essential in the Single Qualification System.

The Audit for the Improvement of the Quality of Health Care encompasses:

- Carry out evaluation, monitoring and improvement activities of processes established as essential.
- Compare the Observed Quality against the Expected Quality, which should have been previously defined by means of technical, scientific and

administrative guidelines and standards.

• The adoption by the institutions of measures aimed at correcting the deviations found in relation to the parameters previously established and at continuing to maintain the conditions of improvement achieved.

The audit for the improvement of the quality of health care must be applied with the health and integrity of the user as the first rule and at no time may the auditor put the life or integrity of the user at risk with his or her gloss.

The particularities of the Medical Audit, according to Colombian legislation, are clarified by a communication from the National Health Superintendence, the Ministry of Health, and the General Directorate of Health System Control (Dirección General de Control del Sistema de Salud).

In compliance with the activities of evaluation and improvement of the quality of health care, and until the practice of medical auditing is standardised, professionals practising this discipline are able to apply commonly accepted auditing methods.

The working papers created during the audit work are part of the quality reports and shall be submitted when requested by the competent authorities in the course of investigations and surveillance and control actions.

The aforementioned communication adds in relation to this issue and in accordance with the above, that the Directorate considers that the administering entities can make use of generally accepted auditing procedures and techniques, but these should generally be carried out with the aim of measuring the care provided to users and to be able to create processes for improvement.

With regard to the pertinence of the management and treatment ordered, the Management considers that the Medical Auditors must maintain the criteria of the treating physicians who are exercising their healthcare services in a direct manner to the patient and who direct their management according to their scientific knowledge, their experience, the management guides or protocols implemented in the institution, the clinical situations of the patient, among other elements. These allegations are of the medical act as such and the differences found between colleagues should be clarified by the Colombian Medical Federation in accordance with the provisions of Article 31 of Law 23 of the year 1981 and not be these factors to gloss the accounts.

How to Design an Audit Programme

1. Planning, it is necessary to structure an audit plan, which should have at least the following sections:

- The scope
- The scope of the audit

- The timeliness of implementation
- Priority processes
- The audit team
- The lead auditor
- Guides, standards, manuals
- Design the formats
- Inform the person responsible for the process to be audited of the start date of the audit.

2. In developing the audit, the following steps are a guide for the execution of the audit:

- Report to the official in charge of the area.
- Explain the procedure to be carried out, collect information using statistical reports, data, figures, fill in audit forms.
- Follow up day-to-day activities by analysing performance, involve here all those responsible for important processes to take an active part in the SELF-CONTROL Process.
- To collect indicators, identifying risk factors (adverse events).
- Design a format to record the results obtained, with conclusions and recommendations.

3. Make recommendations.

- Highlight the strengths found.
- Stimulate self-control behaviour.
- Clearly identify the non-conformities found
- Communicate process deviations to all those involved in the detection of the event.
- Inform management of the obligation for an improvement plan.

4. Follow-up, follow-up actions should be scheduled, such as:

- The improvement plans
- To interventions resulting from audit recommendations
- To the implementation of corrective and preventive actions
- The indicators assessed

For a comprehensive audit process, a multidisciplinary team must be in place, led by a lead auditor who will prioritise the important processes and the action plan to be implemented by the audit team.

1. Review whether the institution complies with the standards of the habilitation process. HABILITATION provides security to the user, as they are treated in institutions that comply with established standards, which are strictly structural, but which must be complied with.
2. If the institution complies with 100% of the standards of the accreditation

process, it must continue with the work of achieving ACCREDITATION, which goes beyond compliance with the minimum requirements, it goes to the processes and to trying to improve them, to continuous planning where the only beneficiary must be the user, all circumscribed to the model of continuous improvement, motivating the culture of self-control, of organisational growth where all the staff of the organisation are included with their constant recognition of their talent, competitiveness and sustained training within their process and with those with whom they are related. Accreditation is nothing more than a method of preventing complications.

3. The audit should be a stable and methodical process of monitoring the organisational processes that have been previously stipulated as the main ones, i.e. those that have to do with the direct care of the user from the moment he/she enters until he/she leaves the process that provided the care, fulfilling all his/her perspectives. It should contain the following tasks depending on the internal organisation of the audit process.

- Pre-invoicing audit
- Response to glosses
- Evaluation of Clinical Practice Guidelines
- Control of Variance of the application of Clinical Practice Guidelines and Care Protocols.
- Sentinel Events Programmes
- Adverse Events Programmes
- Institutional Mortality Probably Avoidable
- Preventable Maternal and Perinatal Mortality
- Preventable Adverse Drug Events
- Hospital Stay Utilisation Review Protocol
- Cancellation of Surgeries
- Patient Monitoring for Chronic Consultation
- Assessing the Adequacy of Medicines Utilisation
- Evaluation of Waiting List Management
- User Satisfaction Surveys (including analysis of perceptions vs. expectations)
- Focus groups
- Petitions, Complaints and Grievances Systems

4. Include the evaluation of standardised, mandatory hospital committees that can be applied according to the type of entity.

- Hospital Ethics Committee
- Transplant Committee
- Committee on Infection, Prophylaxis and Antibiotic Policy

- Pharmacy and Therapeutics Committee
- Epidemiological Surveillance Committee
- Technical - Scientific Committee
- Blood Bank Committee
- Teaching and Research Committee
- Medical History Committee
- Emergency Committee

Chapter 12

Decision-Making Tools

A good decision is based on knowledge and not on numbers.

Plato

Today's management requires fast decision making, this is reflected in the opportunity cost, a manager must be fully confident about the tools he or she can employ for decision making.

The mechanisms recommended for decision-making in adopting the PLECOSER model are not exclusive of other mechanisms or models developed, but these concepts can easily lead to the development of efficient management systems.

Mechanisms to assist decision-making:

- Checklists
- Working Committees
- Pareto chart
- Spider Diagram

There are many more mechanisms, but these are recommended because they are simple to apply and can be used at different stages of the management process.

Checklists

The checklist is a mechanism that helps to establish the development of the process and the fulfilment of tasks.

When should it be used?

The checklist can be used at any time when it is necessary to ensure that all necessary steps or actions have been taken in data management and decision making.

Why do the checklist?

1. Determine the purpose of the data being collected.
2. Define the type of data required.
3. Identify where data should be collected.
4. Identify from whom data should be collected.
5. Determine whether data are available.
6. Determine the methods to be used to collect the data.
7. Determine how much data needs to be collected.
8. Decide who collects the data.
9. Determine the time period.
10. Decide how the data will be analysed.

- Control charts
- Histograms

- Pareto chart
- Review sheet

11. Ask good questions. Information questions should be focused and precise.
12. Audit the collection process, validate data.

Working Committee

The relationship between the staff of an organisation can be realised through individual work and/or teamwork; in the second condition, communication is necessary to meet and make decisions.

Working committees, how to develop them:

- Send the agenda and important information in advance of the meeting. Gather all the information necessary for decision-making in advance of the meeting and send the information to the person responsible for coordinating the activities to be discussed; if there is anything that needs to be done to prepare and decide, hold separate meetings and telephone or personal conferences to understand and learn about new ideas and/or difficulties to be discussed at the next meeting; define the information to be taken away for study, justification.
- Issue the work agenda.
- Define the purpose of the meeting.
- Limit attendance at the meeting. Only as many people as necessary should be present.
- Plan the time of the meeting. The meeting should be designed to meet the objectives of the meeting; it should last only as long as scheduled.
- Define the responsibility of each participant. Define the activities to be dealt with, indicating the persons who will be responsible for coordinating them.
- Define the place, date and time of the meeting.
- Establish concrete activities and time limits to cover them.

For the committee to be successful it must:

- Start the meeting at the stipulated time. Do not wait for late arrivals, as this will punish those who are punctual.
- Assign a minute taker, coordinate time and be specific in discussing the items to be discussed.
- Coordinate activities through the agenda and do not get distracted from it.
- Avoid interruptions. Questions at the end
- Evaluate the main points arising from the meeting.
- At the end of the meeting, finalise the conclusions.
- Finish on time.

Post-committee:

- Draft the minutes of the meeting. Include in the minutes the decisions, persons responsible for coordinating the activities arising from the meeting and set commitment dates. Once the minutes are available, distribute them no later than 72 hours after the end of the meeting.
- Follow-up. The person responsible for the meeting should follow up on the progress and results of the agreements reached at the meeting.
- Take an inventory of the meetings you attend and assess whether they are productive; if you are the one who should attend, you should use the information to improve your own performance.

Pareto chart

In the early 20th century, Vilfredo Pareto (1848-1923), an Italian economist, conducted research on wealth and poverty. He found that 20% of the people controlled 80% of the wealth in Italy. Pareto in his subsequent studies observed many other similar distributions. In the early 1950s, Dr. Joseph Juran found evidence for *8020* distributions in a wide variety of situations. In particular, the event seemed to be found without deviation in quality-related problems. A common phrase for the 80/20 rule is that it comes from "80% of our business comes from 20% of our customers".

Therefore, PARETO ANALYSIS is a formula that separates the "vital few" from the "trivial many". A Pareto Chart is used to graphically separate the important aspects of a problem from the unimportant so that a team knows where to direct its efforts to improve. Reducing the most important problems (the highest bars on a Pareto Chart) will be more helpful for overall improvement than trying to reduce the minor ones. On a regular basis, for one issue, 80% of the problems will fall. For the remaining issues, between 2 and 3 issues will be responsible for 80% of the problems.

The Pareto Chart can be used in the following situations:

- When there is a need to draw attention to problems or causes in a methodical way.
- When analysing the different data sets.
- By looking for the root causes of problems and establishing the importance of solutions.
- Where data can be classified into categories.

Pareto is a widely used method for data analysis and therefore practical in the search for root cause during a problem-solving effort. It allows to observe which problems are of major relevance by giving groups the opportunity to place priorities. In frequent cases, a few are responsible for a large part of the negative impact on quality. By focusing attention on these important few, we can achieve the greatest possible gain from our efforts to improve quality.

A team can use the Pareto Chart for several purposes:

- To study the results.
- To plan for continuous improvement.
- Pareto charts are especially valuable as "before and after" pictures to demonstrate what progress has been made. As such, the Pareto Chart is a simple but powerful analysis tool.

The following steps are used to perform the Pareto method:

1. Select logical categories for the identified topic of analysis.
2. Collect data.
3. Order the data from the highest category to the lowest.
4. Total the data for all categories.
5. Compute the percentage of the total that each category represents.
6. Draw the horizontal and vertical axes on graph paper.
7. Plot the scale of the left vertical axes for frequency.
8. From left to right, draw a bar for each category in descending order.
9. Plot the cumulative percentage line showing the portion of the total that each problem category represents.

- On the right vertical axis, opposite the raw data on the left vertical axis, record 100% at the front of the total number and 50% at the midpoint.

10. Plot the cumulative percentage line.

- Starting with the highest category, place a dot in the top right corner of the bar.
- Add the total of the next category to the first and place a dot above the bar showing the cumulative percentage. Connect the dots and record the remaining cumulative totals until 100% is reached.

11. Give a title to the chart, add dates when the information was collected and the source of the data.
12. Analyse the graph to determine the *vital few*.

A Pareto Chart is a bar chart that lists the categories in in descending order from left to right.

A team can use a Pareto Chart to:

- Analyse causes
- Study results and plan for continuous improvement

When trying to interpret the Pareto chart, one has to consider that sometimes the data do not indicate a clear distinction between the categories.

This problem manifests itself in one of two ways:

- All bars in a Pareto chart are more or less of the same height.
- It takes more than half of the categories to add up to more than 60% of the quality defect.

In either event, it would appear that the Pareto principle does not apply. Since the Pareto principle has been shown to be valid in literally thousands of events, it would be highly unlikely that an exception would have been found. It is much more likely that an appropriate breakdown of categories has simply not been chosen. In this case it is necessary to stratify the data in a different way and repeat the Pareto Analysis again. The percentages may never be accurate, but the groups generally get that most of the problems come from only a few carefully stratified difficulties.

Radar Chart (Spider Diagram)

A Spider Diagram is a valuable tool to graphically show the changes between the current state and the ideal state.

A Radar Chart is used to:

- Visually present the changes between the current state and the ideal state.
- Show changes in the strengths or weaknesses of the team or organisation.
- Clearly present important categories of performance.

It is important to use it:

1. Forming the team.
2. Verify the data to be represented.
3. Define rating categories (no more than 10 and no less than 4).
4. Construct the Radar Graph:

- Draw a circle with as many radii as there are categories.
- Write each title at the end of each radius around the perimeter of the circle.
- Number the radii from 0 (lowest) to 10 (highest) starting with zero at the centre of the circle and ending with 10 at the perimeter.

5. Qualify all categories:

- Each team member can rate where they feel the organisation or team is currently at.
- This can be done silently using adhesive dots.

6. The team can develop a team score either by consensus or by calculating an average of the individual scores.
7. Define the team qualification for each category.
8. Interpret and use the results to improve.
9. Indicate the date on the Radar Chart.

Indicators

When implementing the PLECOSER model, quantitative expression of the variables under evaluation is required. This improves knowledge about the behaviour of an organisation or administrative or care area, and this data, when compared with a reference standard, can indicate the deviations of what is evaluated in relation to what was structured in the planning of the system. Indicators are nothing more than quantitative expressions that make it possible to analyse the company or unit, in the areas of efficiency, compliance with programmed activities, user satisfaction, etc.

Characteristics of the Indicators

- Denomination. The designation should refer only to the characteristic or data being measured.
- Purpose of an indicator. This is the purpose for which the selected indicator is to be generated.

Reference Levels

The act of measuring seeks to compare and this is not possible without a reference against which to examine the value of an indicator.

There are different reference levels:

- Historical level. It is found from the analysis of a time series of an indicator, presenting how it has changed over time with that information and applying the techniques of analysis and projection.

Technical level. The maximum level of production possible with a given technology, inputs, labour and working methods.

Information System

The information system must ensure that the data collected for the generation of indicators is timely, reliable and accurate so that rational and effective decisions can be made.

Information System Principles

- Gradualness. Information to be delivered to be developed and implemented in a phased manner.
- Simplicity. Information shall be delivered in such a way that its content is fully understood.
- Focus. Information will be focused on disseminating the main concepts related to decision-making processes.
- Validity and reliability. The information will be valid in the sense that it positively shows central and reliable topics in relation to the measurement of the event at all stages.
- Efficiency. Only information relevant for evaluation and improvement should be selected.

For each indicator it is necessary to define:

- Who reports it
- To whom you report it
- How often to report

Table 5. Characteristics of the Indicators

Indicator Name	Name that identifies the state of the characteristic or event to be monitored. The name should be expressed as specifically as possible, avoiding including causes and solutions in the relationship. Example: Number of Emergencies % referrals made
Purpose	Measures a fact or characteristic.
Decision-maker	For whom? indicator occurs manager, board of directors
Interpretation	What does it mean?
Periodicity	How often to measure. Daily, weekly, monthly, six-monthly, yearly, yearly
Source of data	Name of the document or format, in which the required data is entered
Responsible for generating the data	The unit and position of the person responsible for data collection and information flow to the person responsible for generating the indicator.
Responsible for generating the indicator	Unit and position of the person responsible for the generation and transmission of the indicator to decision-makers.

Table 6. Some examples of IPS Indicators

Of Opportunity	- Timeliness of appointment to the General Practitioner's Office - Timeliness of appointment allocation to the Specialised Medical Consultation - Proportion of cancellation of scheduled surgery - Timeliness of care in emergency consultations - Timeliness of care in imaging services
	- Timeliness of care in general dentistry consultations - Timeliness of scheduled surgery
From Quality Technique	- Re-admission rate of hospitalised patients - Proportion of high blood pressure under control
From Risk Management	- In-hospital mortality rate after 48 hours - Intra-Hospital Infection Rate - Proportion of Adverse Event Surveillance
Of Satisfaction	- Overall Satisfaction Rate

Source: Author's elaboration

Table 7. Some examples of EAPB indicators

From	- Timeliness of appointment allocation in General Medical

Opportunity	Consultation - Timeliness of appointment allocation at the Consultation Medical Specialist - Number of tutelas due to non-provision of POS or POS-S services - Timeliness of POS Drug Delivery - Timeliness of scheduled surgery - Timeliness of appointment scheduling in general dentistry consultations - Timeliness of care in imaging services - Timeliness of referral in the EAPB
Quality Technique	- Proportion of adequate immunisation schedules in children under one year of age - Timeliness of cervical cancer screening
Risk Management	- Pneumonia Mortality Rate in High Risk Groups - Maternal Mortality Ratio
From Satisfaction	- Overall Satisfaction Rate - Proportion of complaints resolved within 15 days - Transfer rate from EAPB

Source: Author's elaboration

Recommended Indicators for IPS

TOTAL MORTALITY RATE

• Definition. Proportion of discharges due to death in relation to the total number of patients discharged, in a given period.

• Interpretation. This is an indirect measure of the hospital institution's capacity to respond, which means that it has to do with the management of resources for the care of the population to be attended as well as with the technical-scientific capacity offered.

• Scope. This hospital mortality rate needs to be studied with other aspects that have to do with the previous health conditions of the patient and the pathology itself.

• Methodology.

$$\frac{\textit{Número de egresos por muerte}}{\textit{Número total de egresos}} x\ 100$$

Number of discharges due to death

Total number of discharges

• Source. Institutional statistics.

• Reporting periodicity. Monthly.

MORTALITY DURING THE FIRST 24 HOURS IN EMERGENCY CARE

• Definition. Proportion of patients discharged due to death during the first 24 hours of their care in the emergency department, with respect to the total number of patients attended in that department during the period.

• Interpretation. It is an indirect measure of the institution's response capacity in the emergency department.

• Scope. In addition to the indications for the interpretation of the general mortality indicator, other aspects must be taken into account for emergency care that have to do with the severity of the clinical cases attended (Triage Classification), the patient's previous emergency care and the availability of a referral system.

• Methodology.

$$\frac{\begin{array}{c}\textit{Número de egresos por muerte en las primeras 24 horas,}\\ \textit{de pacientes ingresados por urgencias}\end{array}}{\textit{Número total de pacientes ingresados al servicio de Urgencias}} x\ 100$$

$$\frac{\begin{array}{c}\textit{Number of discharges due to death in the first 24 hours,}\\ \textit{of patients admitted for emergencies}\end{array}}{\textit{Total number of patients admitted to the Emergency Department}}$$

• Source. Institutional statistics.

• Frequency. Monthly.

• Remarks. A record should be kept of patients admitted to the Emergency Department. In addition, include data on patients who are referred to other services.

HOSPITAL-ACQUIRED INFECTIONS

• Definition. The proportion of patients who acquired infection within the institution.

• Interpretation. Hospital-acquired infections are an indirect measure of some quality characteristics that have to do on the one hand with safety as a reduction in the risk of acquiring an infection in the hospital environment, as the institution has the minimum requirements of structure and processes aimed at this end, such as biosecurity measures, in accordance with the complexity and volume of the activity carried out. The scientific technical rationality that has to do with the use of management guidelines for specific clinical entities such as surgery in septic patients, antibiotic therapy, follow-up protocols for nosocomial infections.

• Scope. It is necessary to take into account other variables such as the pathology itself, the complexity and specialisation of the institution providing the services.

- Methodology.

$$\frac{\textit{Número de infecciones intrahospitalarias}}{\textit{Número total de egresos}} x\ 100$$

Number of nosocomial infections
Total number of outflows

- Source. Institutional statistics.
- Periodicity. Reports shall be monthly.

WAITING TIME TO ACCESS A SERVICE

- Definition. The response time in current days that elapses between the date of request for services from a provider institution and the actual delivery of services.
- Interpretation. The measurement of waiting time translates the response time of the hospital institution to the demand for services and reflects the accessibility and timeliness of the services provided by the service provider institution.
- Scope. One of the limitations is the supply of services in some regions.
- Methodology.

General Consultation. Days of the General Consultation - day of the appointment request.

Specialised Outpatient Consultation. Day on which the specialist consultation is carried out - day on which it is requested.

Elective surgery. Day of scheduled surgery - day of request for surgery scheduling.

- Source. Consultation records and surgery records.
- Periodicity. The cut-off for the calculation of these response times must be done every month end.

RE-ADMISSION TO THE EMERGENCY DEPARTMENT (LESS THAN 72 HOURS)

- Definition. Re-admission or readmission of patients to the emergency department within 72 hours of discharge.
- Interpretation. This indicator will give us an account of the quality of care in terms of the technical-scientific rationality and effectiveness of the diagnosis and treatment applied in patient care, as well as the institution's capacity for resolution in patient education.
- Scope. Follow-up of the treatment imposed by the treating physician and self-care. As for possible biases in the measurement, there will be users who may re-enter another provider institution and so far we are not able to capture this information.

- Methodology.

Number of re-admissions to the emergency department in less than 72 hours

---X
100
Total number of patients registered in the Emergency Department

- Source. Statistical data from the emergency department.
- Frequency: monthly.

PERCENTAGE OF POST-SURGICAL PATIENTS RE-ADMITTED IN THE FIRST MONTH

- Definition. Proportion of re-entry or readmission of patients to the health care institution, up to one month after discharge, of patients who have undergone a surgical intervention.
- Interpretation. This indicator will give us an account of the quality of care in terms of technical and scientific rationality as well as continuity and comprehensiveness of patient care.
- Limits of interpretation. Follow-up of the treatment imposed by the treating physician. In terms of possible biases in the measurement, there will be users who may be re-admitted to another provider institution and so far we are not able to capture this information.
- Method of calculation.

$$\frac{\textit{Número de reingresos al servicio de urgencias en menos de 72 horas}}{\textit{Número total de pacientes registrados en el servicio de urgencias}} x\ 100$$

Number *of post-surgical patient readmissions within one month of discharge*
Total number of surgical discharges

- Source. Institutional statistics.
- Frequency. Monthly.

THE SENTINEL EVENT

The sentinel event indicator designates all adverse events or complications occurring during health care, which are more attributable to health care than to the underlying disease and which may lead to death, disability or deterioration in the patient's health status, delayed discharge or prolonged length of stay in hospital.

Some examples:

- Suicide of a hospitalised psychiatric patient
- Unscheduled admission to the ICU after a procedure involving the administration of anaesthesia
- Patients with bronchoaspirative pneumonia in paediatrics or neonatal ICU
- Patients with positional ulcers
- Inadvertent dystocia
- Postpartum hypovolemic shock
- Mothers with in-hospital seizures

- Surgery on the wrong part or on the wrong patient
- Patients with severe hypotension post-surgery
- Patients with infarction within 72 hours post-surgery
- Readmission to hospital for the same cause within 15 days
- Surgeries or procedures cancelled due to factors attributable to organisational or practitioner performance
- Patients with deep vein thrombosis who are not monitored for coagulation tests
- Readmission to the emergency department for the same cause within 72 hours.
- Wrong delivery of a neonate
- Intra-institutional child stealing
- Leakage of inpatient psychiatric patients
- Intra-institutional use of psychoactive substances
- Foreign body retention in hospitalised patients
- Burns from phototherapy lamps
- Premature rupture of membranes without defined conduct
- Revision of joint replacements due to late start of rehabilitation
- Post-surgical dislocation in hip replacements
- Post-transfusion accidents
- Mechanical ventilation pneumothorax
- Perinatal asphyxia
- Deterioration of the patient's Glasgow Classification on the Glasgow scale without treatment
- Post-resuscitation sequelae

Sentinel events at the insurer

- Tutelas for non-provision of POS services
- Duplicate affiliates
- Complaints about non-provision of POS services
- Patients dissatisfied with what they see as unjustified barriers to accessing care
- Request for transfer before the legal minimum period
- Patients who die while on the waiting list for authorisation or performance of a diagnostic aid or disease-related procedure.
- Complications attributable to non-availability of supplies or medicines
- Patient complications or failures in continuity of treatment attributable to long waiting times
- Delays in the supply of inputs or medicines due to administrative procedures.

Chapter 13

Occupational Health and Safety Management System

Working safely is like breathing: if you don't, you die Jerry Smith

Within the bases of the PLECOSER model, the occupational health and safety management system is a sample to follow of the management system, which aims to anticipate, recognise, evaluate and control occupational risks that may affect occupational health and safety. So it is prudent to analyse Resolution 0312 of 2019 which repeals Resolution 1111 of 2017, where the minimum standards for the Occupational Safety and Health Management System and the implementation of the OSHMS of a company are established.

In addition to promoting a culture of occupational risk prevention in which all actors in the system actively participate, including all employees regardless of how they are hired, this regulation is used for the management and implementation of the PLECOSER model. In this way, SG-SST provides companies, including health service providers, with a logical, step-by-step process based on continuous improvement that allows:

- Preventing accidents at work and occupational diseases
- Protect and promote workers' health

The minimum standards of the OSHMS are a group of rules, requirements and procedures that are mandatory for employers and contractors. By means of which it is possible to establish, examine and control the minimum conditions of technical-administrative capacity and financial and patrimonial sufficiency that are essential for the functioning and development of the OSHMS.

The field of application and coverage of the OSHMS is all persons related to the following areas: - The field of application and coverage of the OSHMS is all persons related to the following areas:

- Public and private employers
- Recruiters of personnel under civil, commercial or administrative contracts, among others.
- Solidarity economy and cooperative sector organisations
- Associations or associations that affiliate self-employed workers
- Temporary service companies
- Students affiliated to the occupational risk management system and workers on assignment.

The basic standards for OSHMS according to the classification of companies and their size.

Table 8. Classification of Companies according to number of workers and risk

Companies	Risk class	Requirements to be

		met (number of standards)
10 or less workers	I, II and III	7
From 11 to 50 employees	I, II and III	21
Agricultural production units (up to 50 workers)	I, II and III	3
More than 50 workers	I, II, III, IV and V	60
Any number of workers	IV and V	60

The basic OSHMS implementation standards for smaller companies were designed after learning of the unfeasibility of fully implementing Resolution 1111 of 2017 on occupational health in Colombia.

Since this standard established more than 100 requirements (each standard could contain in some cases more than 3 requirements) for the implementation of the OSHMS, many of which were actually innocuous for effective preventive management, it was necessary to create Resolution 0312 of 2019.

The new Resolution 0312 of 2019 on occupational health in Colombia is part of a group of government decisions aimed at facilitating and streamlining the regulations that companies must comply with in order to operate.

The ultimate objective of the implementation of the OSHMS and the 7 basic standards of Resolution 0312 of 2019 is to help a large percentage of companies that are part of the economic factor of the country, which is made up of medium and small enterprises (MSMEs), to be prepared favourably, being reliable in terms of welfare, safety and health at work.

Being able to manage your variables under the application of the PLECOSER model, i.e. putting into practice each of the requested topics, will lead to a culture of prevention rather than reaction, demonstrating confidence in the business relationship.

The amendments to the standard help the rapid adoption of the total number of standards covered by Resolution 0312 of 2019, it could be argued that in reality more than 100 requirements for the implementation of OSHMS expire, which in smaller companies or in the agricultural sector would be difficult to comply with due to the business model of their activity.

Table 9. The 7 standards of Resolution 0312 of 2019

Standard No.	Definition
1°	Designer of the management system (technician, technologist, university graduate, specialist), which involves demonstrating the

	designer's assignment by means of a letter or minutes, in addition to his or her professional certifications. It is not necessary to hire a person, but the employer must be sure that he has solid technical support to meet all the requirements of the process in terms of health and safety at work.
2°	Support for payment to the integral social security system (health, pensions and labour risks). This indicates that the trust that customers may have when contracting a company ranges from the quality of the product, timeliness of delivery, and even the welfare of all the staff involved in the production chain and / or marketed service, generating a real bond of trust in whoever contracts or buys.
3°	Training programme, for which there should be, at a minimum, a timetable and a format for registering signatures. Although resolution 0312 on occupational health in Colombia does not establish it, a company can voluntarily create a document that allows for the evaluation of each training. The content of the training programme or plan, as it is often called, would be expected to meet the expectation of providing guidance on the priority risk that has arisen in the company, in order to assess the administrative controls to be implemented.
Standard No.	**Definition**
	The aim is to develop the soft competences of the human factor in the company and to ensure that these competences can be the footprint that is reflected in the safe behaviour of all personnel during the development of their activity.
4°	Annual work plan, which, as defined in Decree 1072 of 2015, must be signed by the legal representative. It is important to underline that the work plan should be reviewed at every new period, i.e. year by year. It is not possible to start each time as if it were the first time, but on the contrary, for each period the objectives must evolve to show the maturity of the Occupational Health and Safety Management System. It includes, of course, innovation and the application of new strategies and technologies that contribute to the prevention of adverse events, whether accidents or occupational diseases.
5°	Occupational medical evaluations, which, as defined in the

	regulations in force, must respond to a *job profile* which must include, in addition to their functions, the person's own requirements in terms of competencies and skills. This document is evaluated by the doctor in conjunction with the matrix for hazard identification, risk assessment and evaluation in order to issue the profesiogramme, which constitutes the guide for the medical centre to orientate itself about the physical and laboratory tests to be applied to the applicant or the worker, as applicable if it is a periodic occupational medical examination. Resolution 0312 of 2019 on occupational health in Colombia does not define it, but it is important to submit a letter with the medical recommendations issued by the evaluating physician for the
Standard No.	**Definition**
	follow-up by the company of the worker who must be medically monitored.
6°	Hazard Identification, Evaluation and Risk Assessment (HHRA). The right thing to comply with this standard requested by Resolution 0312 of the year 2019 for the adoption of the OSHMS of a company, is to have a documented procedure that defines those responsible, methodology, evaluation and assessment criteria, etc., which helps anyone with the necessary knowledge to execute without difficulty the appropriate updates every time a change in the processes, building, a serious or fatal accident, occupational disease, among others, appears. In another sense, the hazard identification matrix is an indicator that allows to prioritise the most critical risks in the company and to look for actions that will help to reduce the exposure of the personnel. It is a fully active document. It cannot be left on file and must always be consulted.
7°	This seventh standard is perhaps the most important of all those defined by Resolution 0312 of 2019 for Occupational Health in Colombia for small companies: it is the application of prevention and control measures for all identified hazards and risks. This standard is really open to the preventive needs of any small company, because if the organisation has a risk of heights, it must create a prevention programme against heights.
Standard	**Definition**

No.	
	falls, work permit forms, risk analysis forms, etc. In the case of companies with mechanical risk, they must document the mechanical risk programme, the blocking and labelling programme; if the company has a biomechanical risk, it must carry out the risk assessment with the support of the physiotherapist or ergonomist; if the company handles chemicals, it must comply with the chemical risk regulations; it must label using a globally harmonised system; it must carry out occupational hygiene assessments, among many other activities.

Source: Authors' elaboration

The flexibility and content of standards facilitates, offers easier compliance and verification, and thus, as the company grows and has a larger structure, capital, departments and specialised personnel, will have to apply a large number of standards gradually until completing the 21 standards or members of the OSHMS if they exceed the hiring of 11 to 50 people ordered according to Decree 1607 of 2012 with risk class between I and III or III, until reaching compliance with the total of 62 standards if the company comes to exceed the hiring of 50 or more workers or if it is classified as risk IV or V.

While the standards of the new Resolution 0312 of 2019 are the minimum standards to comply with the Occupational Health and Safety Management System, this means that a small company can voluntarily implement the standards it deems essential according to its activity.

In this way, Resolution 0312 of 2019 is considered a step forward for the gradual implementation of occupational health and safety in small companies, all those that are just starting out, those with small capitals, and as they need to adopt more complex or advanced standards, according to the best world practices in this area.

It is important to note that complying with the 7 standards stipulated in Resolution 0312 of 2019 does not guarantee compliance with all regulations related to occupational risks. Some employers and preventionists mistakenly believe that their only duty in relation to occupational risk management is restricted to complying only with the seven standards stipulated in Resolution 0312 of 2019 on occupational health in Colombia.

But it is in the same Resolution 0312 of 2019, in its Article 23 where it is stipulated that compliance with these seven standards, does not excuse compliance with other rules of occupational hazards, so that the institution or company is subject to have the vigilance of safety and health at work, along

with the committee of coexistence at work, maintain an emergency plan if required by the fire brigade in the corresponding municipality, have the occupational health and safety policy at hand as stipulated in the unified circular of 2004, provide the induction that has to be written as established in the Decree Law 1295 of 1994 and Resolution 2646 of 2008.
The above perhaps demonstrates the need to re-analyse the identification of all standards that may be applicable outside the 7 standards set out in Resolution 0312 of the year 2019 for the adoption of OSHMS, witness such identification, and engage the best qualified, experienced and competent professional persons to enforce such regulations, in order to give compliance before the government, customers, workers and generally speaking of all people who favour an accurate implementation of an occupational safety and health management system and a sensible application of Resolution 0312 of the year 2019.
For all of the above, the company must make its best effort to demonstrate compliance with the basic standards of Resolution 0312 of 2019, starting from the analysis of management indicators that are the sample of the implementation and development of the occupational health and safety management system.

General Health Administration Students' Contribution to this Chapter

Integrated Health Risk Management (IHRM)

It is a transversal strategy of the integrated health care policy, based on the articulation and interaction of the agents of the health system and other sectors to identify, evaluate, measure (from prevention to palliation) and carry out follow-up and monitoring of health risks for all. It anticipates diseases and injuries so that they do not occur or are detected and treated to prevent their progression and consequences. This strategy aims to achieve a better level of health in the population.
The implementation of ISWM in a territory is based on the priorities identified in the Territorial Health Plan, which is the instrument that allows territorial entities to contribute to the achievement of the strategic goals of the ten-year public health plan and the national development plan, among others.
Risk management programmes emerged in response to scientific advances that enabled the quantification of cancer. Over time, risk management programmes have broadened their scope and evolved.
Placing risk management in the cancer framework identifies two moments:
1. Risk before the disease: healthy people exposed to developing cancer due to different factors; biological, genetic, social, environmental, lifestyles, among others.

Prevention focuses on breast self-examination, screening mammograms and prostate antigen screening in men.

2. Risk during the disease: the pathology is already established and is related to the possible outcomes; disappearance of the disease, decrease of the disease, progression, no change or death.

Cancer risk management in Colombia is assessed by indicators. The evaluation of the indicators has a range of compliance classified as high, medium and low; there are 14 indicators for breast cancer and 6 for prostate cancer.

Examples:

Indicator:

proportion of women with breast cancer who underwent TNM stabilisation at CNR.

Result:

The following were considered to have medium compliance: sucre, la guajira, choco, atlántico, Magdalena and meta, the rest had high compliance.

Indicator:

Proportion of patients with TNM-staged prostate cancer.

Result:

Nationally only 72.4% of patients are staged, 13 patients are below this value with figures ranging from 68.8% for Nariño to 33.3% for Casanare.

Questions:

1. **What is the objective of health risk management?**

A. Mitigate or shorten the progression of diseases.

b. Mitigate or shorten the consequences of diseases.

c. a and b are true.

d. None of the above.

2. **How is public health risk classified?**

a. Primary risk and secondary risk.

b. Primary risk, secondary risk and tertiary risk.

c. Primary risk and technical risk.

d. None of the above.

3. **What characteristics are taken into account to form risk groups?**

a. High-cost treatments

b. Highly chronic diseases

c. Priority diseases in public health.

d. All of the above.

4. **The objective of the ISWM strategy is?**

a. The articulation and interaction of health actors.

b. Identify, assess, measure, intervene, follow up and monitor health risks.

c. Achieving a better level of population health, a better user experience during the care process and costs commensurate with the results obtained.

d. None of the above.

5. Why did risk management programmes emerge?

a. They arose to treat illness and trauma.

b. They arose to ensure the quality of life

c. They arose in response to scientific advances that allowed the quantification of cancer.

d. None of the above.

Chapter 14

E-Health

Humans will add value where machines cannot. As AI advances further and further, real intelligence, real empathy and real common sense will be in short supply. New jobs will be based on knowing how to work with machines, but also how to leverage these unique human attributes.

Satya Nadella

E-health, a term that defines the ICTs used in health centres for prevention, diagnosis, treatment, monitoring and health management, helps to strengthen health and brings us closer to the 4Ps of medicine: predictive, preventive, personal and participatory. E-health is a term that encompasses the set of information and communication technologies used as tools in the healthcare environment related to prevention, diagnosis, treatment, monitoring and health management to save resources in healthcare systems and enable them to increase their efficiency.

The World Health Organisation defines e-health as the cost-effective and safe use of information and communication technologies to support health and health-related fields, including health care services, medical surveillance, health information and education, health knowledge and research. Information and communication technologies are presented as an indisputable opportunity to improve the various processes associated with health.

Therefore, in order to achieve perfection in the care provided by the health sector, it is necessary to start from an unbreakable principle, such as the doctor-patient relationship, a very delicate and humane subject in medicine.

Such impressive technological advances in medicine, if not consistently controlled by humans, can turn the doctor-patient relationship into one that is dehumanising and becomes a patient-device relationship. Maintaining and improving the doctor-patient relationship is an inalienable duty of all healthcare personnel, which is an inviolable principle of healthcare practice.

Digital health is a generic concept of the use of information and communication technologies to improve individual or general population health. E-health can be considered a branch within digital health, more related to the computerised treatment of health information, applied to health systems. The dissemination of information and communication technologies (ICTs) in the daily life of every person allows these sources to become a strategic partner for public health, whether in the support to solve or prevent health problems, or to improve access to health systems and services.

The use of the internet and the indiscriminate use of mobile phones in itself allows for a wealth of data about a person's health and social behaviours, including the types of internet searches and keywords used, information shared on social networks, e.g. statuses or tweets, medicines purchased and where purchased, restaurants visited and absences from school or work due to illness, as well as various regular actions.

If used appropriately and ethically, the data stored through the use of new technologies may be able to help expose early warnings and other health care alerts, which would help the public health sector, for example, to detect outbreaks early and track cases with greater certainty, identify food-borne diseases immediately, and improve response time to emergency conditions and disasters by being able to locate harmed people with greater speed.

This includes various healthcare products and services, such as mobile applications, telemedicine, wearable monitoring devices and accessories. It also includes everything related to big data, clinical decision support systems, the Internet of Things or health video games, to name a few.

The implementation of health technologies includes activities to realise these technologies in organisations or processes that are implemented in the health service delivery system. In particular, science promotes the use of proven, effective, efficient and safe technologies, reasonably based on safety, in the operational practice of health services. Therefore, several analytical frameworks and recommendations for implementation research have been published.

To this end, we must start with the integration of e-health elements into healthcare delivery including a feasibility study, which analyses the enabling factors as well as barriers to appropriate inclusion; infrastructural, social or cultural. This phase should be based on specialised research that measures the need to implement the technology at the proposed site or service to promote equitable access to the intervention or technology being developed. The next step is organisational adoption, which means that the mandate of the organisation decides to implement the technology into its processes. Such decisions may be influenced by internal and external policies.

While the implementation stage for e-health refers to adaptation, which involves fine-tuning the organisation's internal processes, in this case, health care processes, as well as training the institution's staff in the application of these technologies in these processes, promoting the adoption of the indispensable digital skills.

While this process of alignment is taking place, it is necessary to carry out certain tests to study the operation of the processes. A crucial measurement or study is that of loyalty, which refers to the investigation of the extent to which an activity was implemented as proposed in a defined plan or implementation protocol, as opposed to the measurement of appropriateness, which deals with the extent to which the plan or mediation is changed by users or staff while the implementation is being executed, in order to meet individual requirements.

Research on the adaptation-acceptance of technology by those involved in the care process includes detailed studies on the quality of technology use and the preference of these individuals.

Feasibility studies, on the other hand, measure the degree to which an impact or technology is sustained or widespread in a health service organisation. As part of this subject, the development of standardised implementation activities can be delegated in order to standardise processes according to the changes involved in the incorporation of new information technologies.

In this regard, the development of standard operating procedures or specific technical compliance procedures should be emphasised and the establishment of a technical monitoring system at this stage should be encouraged.

Finally, coverage is the measure of the population that will benefit from the adoption of the technology relative to its intake.

On the other hand, eHealth can be seen as including several applications that reflect specific working conditions in an integrated way and can be incorporated into experiences in different areas of the public health system. Some studies have established the effectiveness and efficiency (cost-effectiveness) of individual eHealth components.

In response to this situation, the World Health Organisation, the Pan American Health Organisation , the Economic Commission for Latin America and the Caribbean and the Organisation for Economic Cooperation and Development have developed policies to promote the adoption of ICTs in health institutions. Undoubtedly, there are serious challenges for access, implementation and operation of these components, mainly in developing countries, at the micro level between individuals, meso level between health facilities and macro level between countries. In this regard, several studies have highlighted the need to strengthen eHealth policy and simultaneously introduce its different elements into the health system to better take into account social media and networks. In the field of health technology, the text Implementation Science is a set of concepts and tools that facilitate the study of the factors that enable the adoption and optimisation of health technologies based on scientific evidence (cost-effectiveness).

Several analytical concepts have been developed in this regard. What follows is a summary of some of the different elements that make up eHealth, as well as a small part of the financing process for the public and health workers in particular. These ideas were used to propose a conceptual framework approach to examine the implementation of each component of eHealth and its impact on the quality of health service delivery.

Components of e-Health

ICTs are currently considered of utmost importance for the provision of health services, as they are considered important inputs for the integral organisation of health information systems in their different stages of population or health service application. Systems have improved communication between medical professionals, between medical professionals and patients, as well as between patients themselves.

New technologies have improved archiving and information management systems through the digitisation of data contained in administrative processes such as user or patient data, resources (financial, material and human) and health requirements in general (medicines, medical devices, among others).

Fundamentally, they currently exist in the administrative systems of services such as appointment scheduling for health services (digital appointment to medical, dental, psychology, etc.), as well as clinical laboratory and pharmacy services, among the main ones.

Similarly, there has been an evolution in the processes of care at health towards the digitalisation of documents, medical records are transformed into electronic medical records (EHR), medical prescriptions written on paper are converted into electronic prescriptions, and the results of clinical analysis and imaging or radiology change from being analysed and delivered on physical media to being delivered on digital media (Picture Archiving and Communication Systems or PAC).

It is through the development of ICTs that the evolution of remote care systems has been achieved through electronic devices, from the use of telephone systems supported by the Internet, which encompasses a vast set of systems that are included in the concept of telehealth, which means the remote provision of preventive, health promotion or curative services. A broad field within telehealth is telemedicine and its various specialities of care (e.g. teleradiology, telepsychiatry, telerehabilitation, telesurgery, telecardiology, etc.).

This recent technology stands out for its ability to facilitate access to specialised health services for people living in remote areas (rural communities, indigenous or remote populations).

The extensive development of mobile communication technologies such as smartphones and wearable devices (tablets, bracelets, watches or other devices) are used to monitor the activities (physical exercise) or health status of individuals and the monitoring of these events and lifestyles by health professionals for decision-making purposes. These devices or instruments are increasingly used in different areas and are becoming part of the so-called mobile health (m-Health). From this public health perspective, these instruments or devices translate into opportunities to be able to intervene with the population in general contexts such as health promotion or the collection of information on people's habits, behaviours or lifestyles, which becomes a great possibility for the dissemination of upcoming health risk alarms that serve for the development of precise and timely interventions (epidemiological surveillance systems).

It is also indispensable to underline as an integral part of e-Health the Clinical Decision Support Systems (CDSS), secondary devices that can preferentially assist healthcare professionals in making decisions in the course of medical care, resulting in a strong outcome for patient safety. These systems have been unfairly referred to as active knowledge systems that use two or more pieces of patient data to give case-specific advice, or as software or programs created specifically as clinical decision aids where the characteristics of an individual patient are added to a systematised database for the creation of clinical knowledge, in addition to assessments or certain suggestions for the patient are exposed to the clinical staff and/or the patient himself in order to make a decision, although there has been some dispute over what has been widely indicated as the concept of a decision aid, which encompasses other support systems.

There is a wide variety of types in which CDSS are used, depending on the types of events and the degree of realisation and evolution of ICT systems for health services. For this reason, a classification of these systems is indicated based on five conditions: the means of use, knowledge and data capabilities, the type of clinical decision support, the way in which information is sent and the system's workload or operation. This part includes software or programmes supported by forms or calculators for decision-making (e.g. renal clearance calculations or scales to assess the patient's health status), as well as specialised software or programmes that automatically identify errors during the prescription stage according to the patient's characteristics.

In addition, another interesting branch of e-Health is the use of electronic media or websites to educate health professionals in health programmes, service users and people in general (e-learning), in order to promote good practice habits when providing health care (health personnel), as well as health promotion or healthy habits (population). In addition, the use of websites translates into an option for patients to optimise the collection of information about their health, empowering them to take part in decisions or to promote communication with other patients (linked to social networks) and thus establish support networks, which would be very important in certain chronic diseases (all these processes are known as e-patient).

ICT for health applications being used in some health systems include:

- Manage the storage, analysis and use of big data for public health, epidemiological surveillance and health promotion and service quality improvement.
- Use of Internet of Things systems to monitor the health and activity of the inpatient or outpatient using internet-connected devices and sensors and follow up therapy management such as medication dosing.
- Machine learning systems to facilitate automated processes and care delivery, improving clinical decision support for diagnosis or treatment of diseases.
- Use of virtual reality or augmented reality technologies for educational, preventive or therapeutic purposes.
- Development of bioinformatics and its application in medicine (biomedical informatics).
- Further development of portable analysis systems, clinical analysis devices or sensors, including mobile computing systems.

It is important to emphasise that the different parts of eHealth offer the opportunity to combine and link across a wide range of activities, which can be opportunities to strengthen health delivery systems.

Currently, there are different ways in which society in general can embrace and appropriate ICTs to be used in health, where two important classes of members can be found: the total population where the users of health services and the health service providers, be they professionals or technicians, are present.

Perhaps in an indirect way, the population can get information on prevention or health promotion through mass media such as television, radio, mobile phone messages or the internet in its different particularities. Furthermore, on the other hand, the population can take over certain parts of e-Health successfully, e.g. research about health information or guidance by using devices such as the telephone (telephone consultation) or the internet. This requires that people overcome the (economic or socio-cultural) barriers to accessing these technologies by deciding to take up these technologies and attain the digital skills required for their use.

The appropriation-incorporation of these technologies by people can be influenced by different elements that can be internal or external. Internal factors may include age, gender, occupation, schooling, socio-economic status and health status; while external factors may include the social environment to which they belong, the development of ICTs in the place where they work, as well as the institutions or health services where they receive care and the effect of the health personnel working in them.

In this case, in order for people who provide their services in the health sector to take advantage of these technologies, the health companies in which they work must overcome the barriers to entry and promote the appropriate application of these technologies among their employees through training in digital skills or abilities. It should be noted that some devices can be used by health professionals voluntarily and freely, such as programmes for smartphones or suitable websites that help in different processes involved in health care. Certain theoretical-conceptual examples have been given to explain the use and enjoyment of these technologies within organisations.

To date, several investigations have been carried out to study and analyse the above-mentioned events.

The acceptance and use of e-Health elements are of preferential use for health professionals, such as electronic medical records, electronic diagnostic systems, image archiving and communication systems, certain clinical decision support systems, telehealth systems used by service providing institutions.

Chapter 15

Knowledge Dissemination

The researcher who does not know what he is looking for will not understand what he finds.

Claude Bernard

During the Covid-19 pandemic, international agencies have sent many messages about the importance of comparing scientific information on health crises. The importance of communicating science is fundamental to meeting the need to improve knowledge. It should be noted that any research conducted must provide accurate results. Therefore, the results obtained in research have no meaning and value if they are not communicated through publication. In addition to scientific reports and the enormous effort to narrow down and harmonise standards, the generation of texts reflecting the results of various scientific fields has also generated great interest and relevance. Humans have been sharing knowledge since ancient times, and there is evidence of writings developed for this purpose before there were standards on how to disseminate scientific knowledge. One of the oldest known scientific works dates back to 300 BC: Euclid's Elements. But it was not until 1946 that the International Organisation for Standardisation (better known as the ISO standard) was born in London. Nowadays, it is very important to clearly define academic texts and their specificities, because only then will the results become an important part of the research field.

The precision, clarity and brevity that characterise documents in a wide variety of forms are also associated with academic expansion. In an academic environment, writing skills and abilities must go well beyond classical syntax or aesthetics, although these subjects are not alien to them, and even fields of study such as the social sciences or humanities allow for greater flexibility. This does not mean that the purpose of texts

The scientific approach should be forgotten or its concepts and methods should be displaced.

To express the above, a communicative purpose is needed, with different edges where all texts meet and how this process is developed professionally in different ways. Among these statements are important identification issues, such as: comparing information, verifying its validity and being able to verify its recommendations or results. Another distinctive issue is objectivity, which is among the first requirements of scientific validity and style placed by the various publications, with a sense of independence from the area of specialisation.

Generality, understood as a property that favours the highest level of understanding by the document's addressees (whether experts or not), should also not be ignored.

In general, these special qualities can be better understood through knowledge and practice of methodical writing skills. Achieving clarity, accuracy, brevity, objectivity and generality does not mean that all available information should be used to complete the text in all circumstances; on the contrary, parameters and filters should be created to help define what is included in the text content, of course, according to the standard citation and bibliography style.

In this way, the writing of articles intended to publish the results of scientific research becomes part of the very task involved in the research process and is indicated as a request to order those results, limiting oneself to what has produced them, as well as the extent of new discoveries or knowledge of such evidence. Undoubtedly, standardisation of format and style is essential not only to clarify one's scope, but also to better implement previous research that supports the findings. In this regard, it is important to allow rules to stand out in writing, in citations and references; such a structure benefits both those developing the text and those who will read it.

The characteristics for the different types of academic texts are presented below.

Different authors, schools and bibliographies formulate a series of texts that are considered academic.

Within the first type of document are the so-called technical notes, defined as short and concise texts, focused on describing changes in techniques or technological processes. Their aim is to focus on the discovery of new solutions, although this does not necessarily mean new contributions or discoveries in the field of research itself. The peculiarity of publications with a technical description is when the author himself comments on his proposal. It is a widely used tool in some fields, however, it is not a type of publication that is generally considered to be a central focus.

Another text with academic dissemination whose main feature is brevity is called Abstract, which is not presented on its own as an independent material, but is part of the organisation of articles, papers, research reports, theses, dissertations and the like, it is defined as an abbreviated description of the subject matter contained in a work, using clear language and a simple and precise wording.

In turn, the synopsis and summary are responsible for presenting content and/or knowledge in a precise and abbreviated manner. These initial formats are usually used more or less frequently, depending on the author's own or institutional dissemination requirements.

Systematic reviews, on the other hand, are responsible for collecting information in relation to a topic and displaying it in an orderly fashion. This format, although not an original publication, has the great advantage of saving a lot of work and time in the technical aspects of obtaining specific information. Its main purpose is to review the literature related to the research topic, contextualise it, critically analyse it and draw conclusions relevant to the research topic. This type of academic writing should be based on an outline style. Of course, synthesis should not be forgotten, but it should show the facet of the analysed topic, so that the central idea put forward by the author is made visible.

The case study, in turn, deals with the in-depth enquiry that takes place in a series of works focused on judging results, research, innovative alternatives and methodological processes in a wide range of fields. It refers to a method with wide application, with an organisation that has a summary, presentation, development, synthesis, conclusion and bibliography.

On the other hand, a technical scientific report is said to act as a reference for an expert in the field or an educated reader to evaluate and/or make recommendations related to the state of the art of the report. problem or process by which a result is achieved. Its elements limit the presentation of this type of informative information in a systematic or chronological order. It generally consists of the following sections: Summary, Introduction, Development, Conclusions and Recommendations, Bibliography and Appendix.

Manuals are also often identified because they serve as an easy proxy for reference searches.

However, due to circumstances, these articles, although also in book form, are more extensive than the handbook and complement their content with a critical approach to the issues they deal with.

Essays, on the other hand, are examples of a certain type of work, the product of research characterised by brevity and in which comments and reflections on the topic of interest are included. However, it is important to clarify that the length of this article is an issue on which not all authors agree, as some articles are published as books, so scientific articles should not be confused with literary articles. The purpose and the language used are the elements that differentiate them significantly. An intrinsic condition related to the essay is its way of arguing about the topic it refers to and the fact that the arguments have to be validated.

Monographs, which according to the established rules are considered more extensive than theses and in some cases are published in a single volume. In addition to being able to analyse a specific aspect, it aims to be able to look at a precise topic in a general and comprehensive way, regardless of the subject or field, with the depth and detail of the more specific elements. For this, two approaches are proposed: interpretative and descriptive, and the scientific accuracy of the methods and techniques used for the analysis must be calculated. If it is a shorter text, it can become an editable article in a professional journal.

On the other hand, the research article is one of the most referenced, used and sought after by institutions and publications, once it is adjusted to certain standardised norms, or through the creation of its own guidelines, such as the possibility of being able to review it on their pages and on current digital platforms.

One of the objectives for this type of academic text is to present an original contribution of knowledge to the theoretical and practical understanding of a subject, to the research advancement of this subject or its application, whether in the scientific, technical or teaching field. Within a standardised structure, which is determined by Introduction, Methods, Results and Discussion (IMRyD), which may vary according to the specific needs directly related to the type of research, the field of study, institutional norms or a particular publication.

A thesis, on the other hand, is a text that contains preparatory work plans and drafts, and is easier to work with when it comes to organising information.

Among them, the wording of the question is very important for this type of text, so it is necessary to analyse and determine the train of thought, depth, time period and specific topic and avoid shortcuts. Solving the problem question. On the other hand, arguments, objectives, assumptions and thematic limitations facilitate the conduct of the research and in most cases form part of the organisation of this type of text.

The second most important issue is the reference system, which includes, among other things, the authors who have published on the topic and the results of previous studies. In addition, the method, timeline, budget and bibliography need to be specified.

It should be noted that, in the elaboration of a thesis, a series of steps must be followed, starting with the search for information, followed by the organisation, writing and style, and the structure and presentation, as the final element of the thesis.

In addition, it is necessary to emphasise the statement of objectives, which form the roadmap to follow in order to provide an answer to the problem, and which within the academic text translate into a guide to the purposes and resources necessary to publish the new knowledge.

Thus, in relation to the field of study, they will be more practical or theoretical, but it should always be borne in mind that the following should be taken into account when writing them: The main condition for them to be achievable, logical and coherent, is that the possibilities and limitations are considered.

There are two questions that will help to make this process a reality: How? and What for? The answer to these two questions will set us on course towards the specific and general objectives accordingly. Clarity in writing them down is of utmost importance.

On the other hand, the objectives will also show the type of knowledge that is sought to be achieved, which is why it is of great importance to formulate them adequately, in other words, with a sense of precision in relation to what is to be expressed.

These objectives have to be precise, avoiding redundancy and long, unclear paragraphs, and always keeping in mind all the elements that are part of the research.

Once the objectives are well written, they give a glimpse of the type of research, whether qualitative or quantitative, and also help to identify how to address the research topic and the purposes of the research.

For this, it is essential that it shows the process and content of the research, as well as the advancement of new knowledge.

It is therefore the clarity and precision of the objectives that lead in turn to the choice of methods and techniques to achieve them.

In a large majority of scientific publications, a lot of importance is given to this section, as this is the part where the authors get to show how they reached their results and the reliability of these results, which are shown in a smaller form in the conclusions.

Thus, this part synthesises the central idea of the text, and the explanation on which it is based.

As a result, there is a need to evaluate what has been raised, indicating the scope and limitations, and at the same time demonstrating new scopes originating from this topic or from new questions.

BIBLIOGRAPHY

Agora (2022). *Ideas. Analysis of presidential candidate Gustavo Petro's health proposal.* https://agoraasuntospublicos.com/analisis-de-la- propuesta-de-salud-del-candidato-presidencial-gustavo-petro/

Barbera, M., Cecagno, D., Seva, A., Heckler, H., López, M., & Soler, L. (2015). Academic training of the professional in health areas and its adequacy to the job position. *Revista Latinoamericana de enfermagem*, 23(3), 404-410.

Bautista-Espinel, G., Ardila-Rincón, N., Castellanos-Peñaloza, J., & Gene-Parada, Y. (2017). Knowledge and importance, that health area professionals have about informed consent applied to health area care acts. *Universidad y Salud*, 19(2), 186-196.

Betancourt, P., & Gonzáles, S. (2020). *Clima organizacional y motivación en enfermeras del hospital nacional Daniel Alcides Carrión, Lima, octubre-2019.* Lima: Norbert Wiener University.

Betancourt, V. (2003). *Scientific communication.* Finlay.

Bustamante, M., M. Lapo, C. Oyarzún and R. Campos (2017). Analysis of the Teacher's Perception in Three Chilean Universities after the Implementation of the Competency-Based Curriculum. *Formación Universitaria*, 10(4), 97-110.

Cancer Today (2020). *Data visualization.* https://gco.iarc.fr/today/home

Ceballos-Vásquez, P., Jara-Rojas, A., Stiepovich-Bertoni, J., Aguilera-Rojas, P., & Vilchez-Barboza, V. (2015). Care management: a social and legal function of Chilean health areas. Áreas de la salud *actual en Costa Rica*, (29), 1-12.

Cevallos, G. (2015). *Manual of scientific writing. The scientific article.* Málaga: Servicios Académicos Intercontinentales Eumed.net. http://www.eumed.net/libros-gratis/2015/1499/index. htm.

Chaves, M., Menezes, M., Cozer, L., & Alves, M. (2010). Professional competencies of nurses: the developing a curriculum method as a possibility to elaborate a pedagogical project. *Global Health Areas*, 9(1), 1-18.

Clavijo, M., Romero, F., & Paniagua, M. (2016). Evolution of training in health areas. *Medwave*, 16(6): e6505.

Dandicourt, T. (2016). Professional competencies for the specialist in community health areas in Cuba. *Revista cubana de áreas de la salud*, 32(1), 16-26.

De Arco-Canoles, O., & Suárez-Calle, Z. (2018). Role of health professionals in the Colombian health system. *Universidad y Salud*, 20(2), 171-182.

Deming, W. E. (1989). *Quality, productivity and competitiveness: the way out of the crisis*. Díaz de Santos.

Donabedian A. (1969). *A Guide to Medical Care Administration. Medical Care Appraisal -Quality and Utilization*. American Public Health Association.
Donabedian, A. (1986). Quality assurance in our health care system. *Quality assurance and utilization review*, 1(1), 6-12.
Donabedian, A. (1966). Evaluating the quality of medical care. *The Milbank memorial fund quarterly*, 44(3), 166-206.
Donabedian, A. (1984). *The quality of medical care, definition and methods of evaluation*. La Prensa Médica Mexicana
Donabedian, A. (2000). Evaluating physician competence. *Bull World Health Organ*, 78(6), 857-860.
Feo, O. (2003). Reflections on globalisation and its impact on workers' health and the environment. *Ciencia, Saudade Coletiva*, 8(4), 887-896.
Flexner A. (1910). Medical Education in the United States and Canada. A Report to the Carnegie Foundation for the advancement of Teaching. *Bulletin of the World Health Organization*, 80, 594-602.
Garavito, M. (2019). *Personal competencies required for the professional practice of psychology*. Duitama: Universidad Nacional, Abierta y a Distancia.
Gates, B. (2022). *How to avoid the next pandemic*.
Gaviria, D. (2009). The evaluation of health care: a disciplinary commitment. *Investigación y educación en Áreas de la salud*, 27(1), 24-33.
Gómez, M., & Laguado, E. (2013). Evaluation Proposal for Formative Practices in Health Areas. *CUIDARTE Journal*, 4(1), 502-509.
González, E. (2007). Stakeholder theory. A bridge for the practical development of business ethics and corporate social responsibility. Veritas. *Journal of philosophy and theology*, 2(17), 205-224.
González-Esteban, M., Ballesteros-Álvaro, A., Crespo-de las Heras, M., & Pérez-Alonso, J. (2016). Effective tele-health interventions in the
Primary care: systematic review. *Evidentia: international journal of evidence-based health care*, (13), 55-56.
Guerrero-Núñez, S., & Cid-Henríquez, P. (2015). A reflection on autonomy and leadership in health areas. *Aquichan*, 15(1), 129-140.
Juran, J. M. (1964). *Managerial breakthrough*. McGraw-Hill.
Juran, J. M. (1988). *Juran on planning for quality*. Free Press.
Kruger, C., Bauer, L., & D'Innocenzo, M. (2017). Use of the conceptual structure of the international classification on patient safety in ethical-disciplinary processes in health areas. *Global Health Areas*, 16(4), 151162.
Latrach-Anmar, C., Febré, N., Deandes, I., Araneda, J., & González, I. (2011). Importance of competencies in the training of health areas. *Aquichán*, 11(3), 305-315.

Llinás Delgado, A. E. (2010). Evaluation of the quality of health care, a first step for the Reform of the System. *Revista Salud Uninorte*, 26(1), 143-154.
Llinás, A. (2006). Manual de auditoría y gestión de calidad en salud: El modelo Plecoser. *Barranquilla: Simón Bolívar University.*
Llinas Delgado, A. E. (2022). Retos de la educación superior después de la pandemia por sars-cov2. Revista Boletín Redipe, 11(11), 177-182. https://doi.org/10.36260/rbr.v11i11.1916
Milos, P., Bórquez, B., & Larraín, A. (2010). Care management" in Chilean legislation: interpretation and scope. *Ciencia y áreas de la salud*, 16(1), 17-29.
Ministry of Health of Colombia (2017). *Modelo Integral de Atención en Salud (MIAS)*. Minsalud
Ministry of Health and Social Protection, Colombia (2016). *Comprehensive Health Care Policy. A health system at the service of the people*. Minsalud.
Ministry of Health and Social Protection of Colombia (2013, 28 May). Resolution 1841 of 2013. Whereby the Ten-Year Public Health Plan 2012-2021 is adopted. Diario Oficial No. 48811. https://www.alcaldiabogota.gov.co/sisjur/normas/Normal.jsp?i=53328
Ministry of Health and Social Protection of Colombia (2016, 25 July). Resolution 3202 of 2016. By which the Methodological Manual for the development and implementation of the Comprehensive Health Care Routes - RIAS is adopted, a group of Comprehensive Health Care Routes developed by the Ministry of Health and Social Protection within the Comprehensive Health Care Policy -PAIS is adopted and other provisions are issued. Official Journal No. 49947.
https://www.minsalud.gov.co/sites/rid/Lists/BibliotecaDigital/RIDE/DE/DIJ/resolucion-3202-de-2016.pdf
Ministry of Health and Social Protection of Colombia (2018). *Gestión Integral del Riesgo en Salud. Perspectiva desde el Aseguramiento en el contexto de la Política de Atención Integral en Salud*. Minsalud.
Ministry of Health and Social Protection of Colombia (2018). *Política Nacional de Talento Humano en Salud: Dirección de Desarrollo del Talento Humano en Salud*. Bogotá: MinSalud.
Ministry of Health and Social Protection of Colombia (1994). *La reforma a la seguridad social en salud*. Volume 1: Background and results. Minsalud
Morfi, R. (2010). Care management in health areas. *Revista cubana de áreas de la salud*, 26(1), 1-2.
Morín, E., Restricted Complexity, General Complexity, *Estudios Journal*, 8(93), 81-135 (2010)
Najman, J.M. (1982). The Definition of Quality and Approaches to its

Assessment - Donabedian, a. *Community Health Studies*, 6, 311-312.
WHO (1986). *Ottawa Charter for Health Promotion.* http://www1.paho.org/spanish/hpp/ottawachartersp.pdf

World Health Organization. (1994). *Making medical practice and medical education more relevant to people's needs: The contribution of the family physician*. WHO.

Pan American Health Organization. (2007). *Renewal of Primary Health Care in the Americas: Position Paper of the Organization*. PAHO.

Paravic, T. (2010). Health areas and globalisation. *Science and Nursing*, 6(1), 9-15.

Passos Nogueira, R. (1997). Perspectives of total quality management in health services. *Serie Paltex Society and Health* 2000.

Pat, L., Cen, W., G., L., Andrade, N., & Ríos, M. (2021). Innovation in healthcare management: transactional vs. transformational leadership to foster a positive organizational climate. *Revista Iberoamericana de Educación e Investigación en Áreas de la salud*, 11(1), 18-26.

Pérez, M., Enrique, J., Carbó, J., & González, F. (2017). Formative assessment in the teaching-learning process. *Edumecentro*, 9(3), 1-20.

Piaget, J. (1980). *The psychogenesis of knowledge and its epistemological significance.* In: Piattelli-Palmarini eds. Language and learning: The debate between Jean Piaget and Noam Chomsky. London; Routledge & Kegan Paul.

Pontón Laverde, G., Galán Morera, R., and Malagón Londoño, G. (2003). *Audit in health for efficient management*. 2 ed. Médica Panamericana

Soto-Fuentes, P., Reynaldos, G. K., Martínez-Santana, D., & Jerez-Yáñez, O. (2014). Competencies for nurses in the field of management and administration: current challenges for the profession. *Aquichan*, 14(1), 79-99.

Trincado, M., & Fernández, C. (1995). Quality in health areas. *Revista cubana de áreas de la salud*, 11(1), 1-2.

Valenzuela-Suazo, S. (2016). The practice of health areas as a focus for reflection. *Aquichan*, 16(4), 415-417.

Vygotsky, L. S. (1986). *Thought and Language. Massachusetts*: The MIT press.

Vyotsky, L. (1978). *Mind in society: The development of higher psychological processes*.

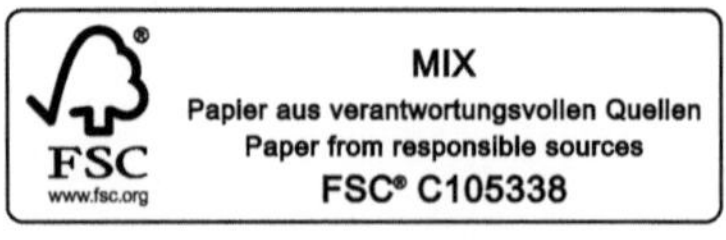

Printed by Books on Demand GmbH, Norderstedt / Germany